Blood and Blood Products:
Safety and Risk

Forum on Blood Safety and Blood Availability

Division of Health Sciences Policy

INSTITUTE OF MEDICINE

Henrik Bendixen, Frederick Manning and Linette Sparacino,
Editors

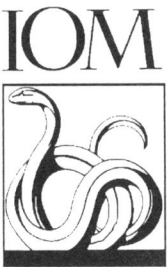

NATIONAL ACADEMY PRESS
Washington, D.C. 1996

National Academy Press • 2101 Constitution Avenue, NW • Washington, DC 20418

NOTICE: The project that oversees this report was approved by the Governing Board of the National Research Council, whose members are drawn from the councils of the National Academy of Science, the National Academy of Engineering, and the Institute of Medicine. The members of the forum responsible for this report were chosen for their special competencies and with regard for appropriate balance.

This report has been reviewed by a group other than the authors according to the procedures approved by a Report Review Committee consisting of members of the National Academy of Sciences, the National Academy of Engineering, and the Institute of Medicine.

The Institute of Medicine was chartered in 1970 by the National Academy of Sciences to enlist distinguished members of the appropriate professions in the examination of policy matters pertaining to the health of the public. In this, the Institute acts under both the Academy's 1863 congressional charter responsibility to be an adviser to the federal government and its own initiative in identifying issues of medical care, research, and education. Dr. Kenneth I. Shine is president of the Institute of Medicine.

Support for this project was provided by the Food and Drug Administration (Contract No. 223-93-1025), Abbott Laboratories, Baxter Health Care Corporation, Ortho Diagnostic Systems, the American Association of Blood Banks, the American Red Cross, the American Blood Resources Association, and the Council of Community Blood Centers. This support does not constitute an endorsement of the views expressed in the report.

Library of Congress Catalog Card No. 96-70494
International Standard Book Number 0-309-05583-0

Additional copies of this report are available from: National Academy Press, Lock Box 285, 2101 Constitution Avenue, N.W., Washington, D.C. 20055.

Call (800) 624-6242 or (202) 334-3313 (in the Washington metropolitan area), or visit the NAP on-line bookstore at **http://www.nap.edu**.

Call (202) 334-2352 for more information on the other activities of the Institute of Medicine, or visit the IOM home page at **http://www.nas.edu/iom**.

Copyright 1996 by the National Academy of Sciences. All rights reserved.
Printed in the United States of America

The serpent has been a symbol of long life, healing, and knowledge among almost all cultures and religions since the beginning of recorded history. The image adopted as a logotype by the Institute of Medicine is based on a relief carving from ancient Greece, now held by the Staatlichemuseen in Berlin.

FORUM ON BLOOD SAFETY AND BLOOD AVAILABILITY

HENRIK H. BENDIXEN, *Chair*, Professor Emeritus, Department of Anesthesiology, Columbia University, New York, New York.
THOMAS F. ZUCK, *Vice Chair*, Professor of Transfusion Medicine, University of Cincinnati, Director, Hoxworth Blood Center, Cincinnati, Ohio
JOHN W. ADAMSON, President, New York Blood Center, New York, New York
ARTHUR L. CAPLAN, Director, Center for Bioethics, University of Pennsylvania, Philadelphia, Pennsylvania
WILLIAM COENEN,* Administrator, Community Blood Center of Greater Kansas City, Kansas City, Missouri
PINYA COHEN, Vice President of Quality Assurance and Regulatory Affairs, NABI, Boca Raton, Florida
EDWARD A. DAUER, Dean Emeritus, College of Law, University of Denver, Denver, Colorado
M. ELAINE EYSTER, Distinguished Professor of Medicine, Division of Hematology, The Milton Hershey Medical Center, Hershey, Pennsylvania
JOSEPH C. FRATANTONI, Director, Division of Hematology, Office of Blood Research and Review, Food and Drug Administration, Rockville, Maryland
HARVEY G. KLEIN, Chief, Department of Transfusion Medicine, Warren Grant Magnuson Clinical Center, National Institutes of Health, Bethesda, Maryland
EVE M. LACKRITZ, Medical Epidemiologist, HIV Seroepidemiology Branch, Division of HIV/AIDS, National Center for Infectious Diseases, Centers for Disease Control and Prevention, Atlanta, Georgia
PAUL R. McCURDY, Director, Blood Resources Program, National Heart, Lung, and Blood Institute, Bethesda, Maryland
PAUL S. RUSSELL, John Homans Professor of Surgery, Massachusetts General Hospital, Boston, Massachusetts
CAPT BRUCE D. RUTHERFORD, MSC, USN, Director, Armed Services Blood Program, Falls Church, Virginia

---

* Served from January 1995 until December 1995.

WILLIAM C. SHERWOOD, Director, Transfusion Services, American Red Cross Blood Services, Philadelphia, Pennsylvania
LINDA STEHLING, Director of Medical Affairs, Blood Systems, Inc., Scottsdale, Arizona
EUGENE TIMM,[**] Member, Board of Directors, American Blood Resources Association, Rochester Hill, Michigan
ROBERT M. WINSLOW, Adjunct Professor of Medicine, University of California-San Diego, and Hematology-Oncology Section, Veterans Affairs Medical Center, San Diego, California

Project Staff

VALERIE P. SETLOW, Director, Health Sciences Policy Division
FREDERICK J. MANNING, Project Director
KIMBERLY KASBERG MARAVIGLIA, Research Associate
MARY JANE BALL, Senior Project Assistant

[**] Served from January 1994 until December 1994.

PRESENTERS

JAMES R. ALLEN, Vice-President, Science, Technology and Public Health Standards, American Medical Association, Chicago, Illinois

HENRIK H. BENDIXEN, Professor Emeritus, Department of Anesthesiology, Columbia University, New York, New York

CARON CHESS, Director, Center for Environmental Communication, Cook College, Rutgers University, New Brunswick, New Jersey

DONALD COLBURN, President and CEO, American Home Care Federation, Enfield, Connecticut, and Member, Blood Products Monitoring Committee, National Hemophilia Foundation

EDWARD A. DAUER, Dean Emeritus, College of Law, University of Denver, Denver, Colorado

BRUCE EVATT, Chief, Hematologic Diseases Branch, Centers for Disease Control and Prevention, Atlanta, Georgia

M. ELAINE EYSTER, Distinguished Professor of Medicine, Division of Hematology, The Milton Hershey Medical Center, Hershey, Pennsylvania

J. MICHAEL FITZMAURICE, Director, Center for Information Technology, Agency for Health Care and Prevention Research, Rockville, Maryland

BERNARD HOROWITZ, Executive Vice-President, Melville Biologics, New York, New York

MASON HOWARD, Chairman of the Board, Colorado Physicians Insurance Company, Greenwood Village, Colorado

HARVEY G. KLEIN, Chief, Department of Transfusion Medicine, Warren Grant Magnuson Clinical Center, National Institutes of Health, Bethesda, Maryland

JAMES J. KORELITZ, Westat, Inc., Rockville, Maryland

EVE M. LACKRITZ, Medical Epidemiologist, HIV Seroepidemiology Branch, Division of HIV/AIDS, National Center for Infectious Diseases, Centers for Disease Control and Prevention, Atlanta, Georgia

JONATHAN D. MORENO, Professor of Pediatrics and Director, Division of Humanities in Medicine, Health Science Center, State University of New York, Brooklyn, New York

M. GRANGER MORGAN, Professor and Department Head, Engineering and Public Policy, Carnegie Mellon University, Pittsburgh, Pennsylvania

KENRAD E. NELSON, Professor and Director, Infectious Diseases Program, School of Hygiene and Public Health, Johns Hopkins University, Baltimore, Maryland

DAVID J. ROTHMAN, Professor of Social Medicine and Director, Center for the Study of Society and Medicine, College of Physicians and Surgeons of Columbia University, New York, New York

ERNEST R. SIMON, Formerly Executive Vice President of Scientific, Medical and Technical Affairs, Blood Systems, Inc., Scottsdale, Arizona

RICHARD K. SPENCE, Director of Surgery, Staten Island University Hospital, Staten Island, New York

SCOTT WETTERHALL, Acting Director for Surveillance & Epidemiology, Epidemiology Program Office, Centers for Disease Control and Prevention, Atlanta, Georgia

THOMAS F. ZUCK, Professor of Transfusion Medicine, University of Cincinnati, Director, Hoxworth Blood Center, Cincinnati, Ohio

Foreword

This is the third in a series of three monographs by the Forum on Blood Safety and Blood Availability. Each monograph provides a review and summary of selected topical presentations at four separate workshops sponsored by the Forum from January 1994 through September 1995. The first volume in the series dealt with the Forum's discussions of governmental regulation of blood banking and was entitled *Blood Banking and Regulation: Procedures, Problems, and Alternatives*. The second volume focused on discussions of availability and was entitled *Blood Donors and the Supply of Blood and Blood Products*. The talks summarized in this document were originally given at workshops on Current Risks of Disease Transmission (July, 1994); Risk and Regulation (January, 1995); and Managing Threats to the Blood Supply (September, 1995). The views expressed, unless otherwise noted, are those of the individual presenters, and do not reflect the views of the individual's employer or the Institute of Medicine. This document is neither a summary of any one workshop nor a comprehensive summary of all of the Forum's workshops. It is a compilation of talks that were specifically selected for their relevance to the issues of safety and risk. To promote full participation by Forum members, presenters, and invited guests, the Forum does not draw conclusions or make recommendations.

The Forum on Blood Safety and Blood Availability was convened by the Institute of Medicine to provide a nonadversarial environment where leaders from the private blood community, the Food and Drug Administration (FDA), academia, and other interested parties could exchange information about blood safety and blood availability, to identify high-priority issues in these areas, and promote problem solving activities such as workshops. Although the inclusion of FDA officials among its members precluded the Forum from offering advice or making recommendations, during its two years of existence, the Forum identified opportunities and problems that are ongoing or expected to arise within the next five years, and has developed approaches to exploiting opportunities or solving problems.

During the final meeting, in September 1995, members of the Forum reviewed its work and addressed the question of how the dialogue that it had fostered might best be continued or improved. One of the questions the group considered was what the criteria should be for any such future venture. Not everyone agreed with everything mentioned, and no votes were taken; consistent with its charter, the Forum reached no specific conclusions or recommendations. The group did, however, request that the collected list of criteria be recorded as a possible starting point for any subsequent initiative. The suggestions on that list included the following "Criteria for a Process of Dialogue:"

1. A consensus oriented procedure capable of reaching closure on the issues being discussed.
2. Participation of diverse constituencies, such as designated representatives of the public.
3. Continuity of people and process, so that issues may be addressed as they arise without the need to fashion a structure and process ad hoc.
4. Conditions supporting openness and candor.
5. Opportunities for discussion in a variety of venues, both public and—where permitted by law—private.
6. Prestigious and neutral, a forum that lends dignity and credibility to the discussions.
7. Expert facilitation, though not necessarily subject-matter expertise, by those who run or manage the process.
8. Less time devoted to education about the issues, allowing more direct engagement with decision-making.
9. Available and ready to be utilized whenever an appropriate issue is identified.
10. Fashioned to be persuasive to Congress and others.

Preface

In its deliberations the Forum has been reminded more than once of the contrast between the remarkable advances in blood safety, a noteworthy achievement by the blood community, and the lack of trust, indeed suspicion, with which that community is viewed, by the public, the media, and those at special risk, all of whom demand further advances in safety. The advances in blood safety to which I refer were reported by several speakers and, subsequently published.[1,2] For example, the risk of HIV, expressed as incidence rates of positive HIV tests in units of donated blood was found by Lackritz to be 1:450,000 to 1:660,000. These ratios reflect the safety of the blood supply, not the risk to the individual recipient, who, after all, is not likely to receive one unit of blood. Data on HIV seroconversion in actual recipients has been reported to be as high as 2:10,000,[3] but unfortunately the data are far too few to have statistical significance. All we know is that the recipient of multiple units of transfusion, such as in open heart or trauma surgery, is at greater risk than is reflected by the per unit blood safety data.

Other areas of medical practice have seen greatly increased safety, e.g., in undergoing surgery and anesthesia. In 1954, a multi-institutional study reported the following death rates caused by surgery 1:420, and death related to anesthesia 1:1,560. About 40 years later one group with a large database reported an anesthesia related mortality among fairly healthy patients having fairly simple surgery as between 1:100,000 and 1:1,000,000, closer to

---

[1]Lackritz EM, GA Satten, J Aberle-Grasse, et al (1995). Estimated risk transmission of the human immunodeficiency virus by screened blood in the United States. *New England Journal of Medicine, 333:* 1721–1725.

[2]Schreiber GB, MP Busch, SH Kleinman, et al (1996). The risk of transfusion-transmitted viral infections. *New England Journal of Medicine, 334*: 1685–1690.

[3]Nelson KE, JG Donahue, A Nunoz, et al (1992). Transmission of retroviruses from seronegative donors by transfusion during cardiac surgery: A multicenter study of HIV 1 and HTLV I/II infections. *Annals of Internal Medicine, 117*: 554–559.

1:1,000,000. An improvement in safety of three orders of magnitude is less than half a decade.[4]

If these advances in safety have not made blood or blood-component transfusion an acceptable risk, we must ask, what is, at any given time, and in any given situation an acceptable risk? Or to ask the often asked question: How safe is safe enough?

To begin to answer this question, a reasonable starting point is a paper of seminal importance, published in 1969 by Starr.[5] His several important contributions began with an explicit differentiation between risks involving voluntary activities, versus risks involving involuntary activities. Starr estimated that individuals will accept voluntary risks, which are three orders of magnitude greater than involuntary risks, not known and agreed to by the individual. Flying a hang glider is highly dangerous, but individuals accept the risk voluntarily, knowingly, feeling in control of their destinies.

Involuntary activities involving risks are often determined by a controlling body, be it a government agency or a leadership group. The persons at risk are not informed, or not fully informed, and they are not part of the decision process.

Starr also offered a baseline for reference; the national death rate from disease, which he calculated to be 1:1,000,000 per person per hour of exposure. He observed that the passenger death rate in commercial aviation was close to this baseline. Today commercial aviation is even safer and is often used as a psychological yardstick to help determine a level of risk acceptability (note that using commercial aviation is in part a voluntary activity, in part the use of a public utility).

Starr further pointed to the effect of potential benefits in making a risk more acceptable; and also the effect of education about risks. Others[6] have pointed out that risk perception is selective and changing, i.e., situational. The transfusion of one unit of blood in a non-life-threatening situation may not be acceptable to the fully informed patient; while multiple transfusions given to the patient undergoing open heart surgery for a life-threatening illness may be readily acceptable to the fully informed patient, who finds the risk of the transfusions small in relation to the risks of surgery and anesthesia. and in relation to what he stands to gain from a cure or amelioration of his heart disease.

---

[4]Eichorn, JH (1989). Prevention of intraoperative accidents and related severe injury through safety monitoring. *Anesthesiology, 70:* 572–577.

[5]Starr C (1969). Social benefit versus technological risk—what is society willing to pay for safety? *Science, 165:* 1232–1238.

[6]Teuber A (1990). Justifying risk. *Journal of the American Academy of Arts and Sciences, 119:* 234–254.

Starr's paper on risk followed by only a few years the paper by Beecher,[7,8] introducing the concept of informed consent. This led to further deliberations in courts of law, in Congress, among ethicists and philosophers, and within the medical professions. In 1982 the first report by the President's Commission, chaired by Morris Abram,[9] concluded that adults are entitled to accept or reject health care interventions on the basis of their personal values and in furtherance of their own personal goals. Also: ". . . ethically valid consent is a process of shared decision making based on mutual respect and participation . . .", and " . . . although the informed consent doctrine has substantial foundation in law, it is essentially an ethical imperative."

Several Forum participants have made reference to both the informed consent doctrine and to the observation that the risk that is known to the risk taker and evaluated in terms of potential gains from taking that risk is often acceptable to the risk taker, making a powerful argument for a public policy of fully informing those at risk, above all those at extra high risk; and involving them in the decision process. There is not always equity in the distribution at risk, and those at special risk must receive special attention.

The Forum has heard repeated references to the need for cost-benefit analysis, and for public policy rationally based on such analysis. To counter the desire for public policy based on cost-benefit analysis stands Teuber,[10] who states that public choices involving risk raise questions of equity to which cost-benefit analysis is blind and about which it has nothing to say. He stresses that potential risk bearers will have to be involved in every stage of the process, in formulating, implementing and adopting public policy.

Speakers and discussants have repeatedly addressed the real and potential problems of so-called look-back, which is a response to the demand that any blood product recipient who received a blood product from a donor subsequently found to be carrying HIV (or other serious pathogens) must be informed of the potential risk. The patient's right to know is recognized, yet the look-back, as conducted in the past, is burdensome and not very

---

[7]Beecher HK, DP Todd (1954). A study of deaths associated with anesthesia and surgery. *Annals of Surgery, 140:* 2–34.

[8]Rothman RJ (1987). Ethics and clinical research: Henry Beecher revisited. *New England Journal of Medicine, 317:* 1195–1199.

[9]President's Commission for the Study of Ethical Problems in Medicine and Biomedical and Behavioral Research (Chair: MB Abram) (1982). *Making Health Care Decisions.* Washington, D.C.: U.S. Government Printing Office.

[10]Teuber A (1990), *op cit.*

effective.[11] In the context of the look-back we also recognize the disparity in technology use between different parts of the blood system. On the one hand, driven by demands for manufacturing safety standards as high as those the pharmaceutical industry is expected to meet, the modern blood center is high technology-dependent, highly computerized and automated. As a result, a look-back is a modest burden for the blood center (i.e., on the donor side). On the other hand, for all but a few medical centers and hospitals, driven less hard by safety standards, a look-back on the patient or recipient side of the system almost invariably has to be done manually, which means that it is labor intensive, expensive and a major burden. This disparity was noted by Simon[12] (see also this volume), who proposes pre-transfusion testing for future transfusion recipients as well as post-transfusion testing, i.e., an ongoing look-back. While ethical issues need resolution, the proposal would fit well in hospital quality improvement programs, which in turn are well suited to automation. Quality improvement programs in most hospitals today are still labor intensive, paper-based and very expensive, however important. Patient care information systems are highly developed in a few hospitals, including quality improvement programs with data being collected automatically and in real time. And the medical record, increasingly, is becoming computer-based, complete with reminders and decision support. Add also that the computer-based medical record is not only readable, but can be read by more than one person at a time.

While the development phase of academic and clinical information system owes much to government support, above all the National Library of Medicine, the growing role of the private sector in health care may further accelerate the development of information systems, as managed care takes hold, with its emphasis on patient education, prevention, and early intervention. The providers will need to know the quality of their product; and the potential for savings is enormous.

Historically, the patient record started as notes scribbled by physicians, strictly for their own use, even today not often shared with a hospital. The hospital record is rarely easy to read, except for the nurses' notes. This record is shared among care providers, but rarely shared with the patient. This exclusion of the patient is changing, as the profession is beginning to recognize that patients are about to become partners in decision making, which

---

[11] Busch MP (1991). Let's look at human immunodeficiency virus look-back before leaping into hepatitis C virus look-back. *Transfusion, 31:* 655–661. Kessler, D and C Bianco (1994). Decreasing efficiency of look-back: implications for HCV. *Transfusion, 34 (suppl):* 54S.

[12] Simon ER (1991). Identification of recipients with hepatitis C and other transfusion transmitted infections: We can do better than look-back. *Transfusion, 31:* 87.

argues that both providers and patients should work from the same database, as suggested as early as 1969 by Weed.[13]

Physicians and hospitals may argue about, who owns the medical record. Legal consideration aside, the medical record should contain little or nothing that is note appropriate for the patient to know. Already physicians are reviewing the patient's record with the patient: on the screen or on a printout. Patients are mostly very appreciative, and this kind of sharing is a road to the building of trust to replace the awe of the old days, and the distrust of more modern times.

The Forum was also reminded that we live in times of assessment and accountability, what Relman[14] called the third revolution in medical care. Prior to about 1965 the physician enjoyed autonomy and independence, alone with God and the patient, and alone with God, when deciding, in loco parentis, how little or how much to tell the patient. In the profession, we are now party to a social contract, within which we accept responsibility to and for each other, and we live with only a modest amount of grumbling about quality assurance, utilization reviews, accreditations and regulations, Congressional hearings, and many other forms of accountability. Paternalism is dead, and we are told that we still pay a price for not having involved the risk bearers more fully in the decision process in the 1980s, when the HIV problems first arose.

Henrik H. Bendixen
Chair, Forum on Blood Safety and Blood Availability

---

[13]Weed LL (1969). *Medical Records, Medical Education and Patient Care*. Chicago: Year Book Medical Publishers, Inc.

[14]Relman AS (1988). Assessment and accountability—the third revolution in medical care. *New England Journal of Medicine, 319:* 1220–1222.

Contents

I **Current Risks of Disease Transmission** 1
Blood and Blood Components: How Safe Are They Today?,
Kenrad E. Nelson, 3
Viral Inactivation of Blood Products: A General Overview,
Bernard Horowitz, 17

II **Guarding the Blood Supply** 25
The Retrovirus Epidemiology Donor Study: Rationale and
Methods, *Thomas F. Zuck*, 27
Demographic and Serologic Characteristics of Volunteer Blood
Donors, *James J. Korelitz*, 31
CDC Surveillance of Donors, *Eve M. Lackritz*, 39
Surveillance of Recipients, *James R. Allen*, 45
CDC Surveillance of High-Risk Recipients, *Bruce Evatt*, 53
CDC Surveillance for Unknown Pathogens, *Scott Wetterhall*, 59

III **New Ideas for Safety and Monitoring** 67
Information Technology and Blood Safety, *J. Michael Fitzmaurice*, 69
Strategies for Dealing with Potentially Infected Recipients,
Ernest R. Simon, 77

IV **Risk Tolerance** 81
Beneficial Aspects of Surgical Transfusion, *Richard K. Spence*, 83
Trade-off of the Risk of Hepatitis and the Benefit of Clotting Factor
Concentrates in the 1970s and 1980s, *M. Elaine Eyster*, 93
Examples of Risks That We Tolerate, *Harvey G. Klein*, 101

V Risk Communication 109
A Mental Model Approach to Risk Communication,
M. Granger Morgan, 111
Risk Communication: Building Credibility, *Caron Chess,* 117
Attitudes Toward Risk: The Right to Know and the Right to Give
Informed Consent, *Jonathan D. Moreno,* 127
Patients, Informed Consent, and the Health Care Team,
David J. Rothman, 143
Communication of Risk and Uncertainty to Patients,
Donald Colburn, 149

VI No-Fault Insurance 155
Administrative and "No-Fault" Systems for Compensating Medically
Related Injuries, *Edward A. Dauer,* 157
The Colorado and Utah Models of Compensating Patient Injury,
Mason Howard, 165

VII Concluding Remarks 175
Henrik H. Bendixen, 177

Appendixes 179
A Acronyms and Abbreviations, 181
B Workshop Participants, 183

Blood and Blood Products:
Safety and Risk

I

Current Risks of Disease Transmission

Blood and Blood Components: How Safe Are They Today?[1]

Kenrad E. Nelson

Control of transfusion-transmitted infections is pretty much of a success story, at least in the United States, although in the rest of the world the problem of transfusion-transmitted human immunodeficiency virus (HIV) and other viruses such as hepatitis C virus (HCV) is still one of some magnitude. I want to review some of the data collected in the United States over the 10 or 12 years since the risk from HIV was recognized, then briefly describe some recent data I have collected in Thailand, and conclude by reviewing my own data and those of others on transmission of hepatitis and other diseases, viral and bacterial.

Blood banks have used three broad strategies to control transfusion related infections. First and most important are efforts to exclude donors whose behaviors might put them at high risk for HIV infection or hepatitis, such as drug users, homosexual or bisexual men, or heterosexuals with high-risk sexual partners. Second is active recruitment of low-risk repeat donors. Seventy to 80 percent of donors in the United States are now repeat donors. Finally, and what the public focuses on most, is serologic screening, which in fact may be the least important of the preventive measures.

A paper published in *Transfusion*[2] by Michael Busch from the Irwin Memorial Blood Bank in San Francisco showed that during the late 1970s and early 1980s, transfusion-transmitted HIV infections in San Francisco were a substantial problem. Busch's estimate is that roughly 5,000 people in San Francisco had transfusion transmitted HIV infections and that more than 2,000 developed acquired immunodeficiency syndrome (AIDS) from transfusions

---

[1]This chapter was originally presented to the Forum in January 1995, but was updated by the author in October 1996 to reflect some important new developments.

[2]Busch, MP, MJ Young, SM Samson, JW Mosley, JW Ward, HA Perkins (1991). Risk of human immunodeficiency virus (HIV) transmission by blood transfusions before the implementation of HIV-1 antibody screening. The Transfusion Safety Study Group. *Transfusion, 31(1):* 4–11.

from a single blood bank. Expressed as prevalence of HIV among donors in 1982 and 1983, more than 1 percent of all donors were HIV positive. However, long before screening was begun in 1985, this had been reduced six- or sevenfold by excluding donors who had a history of male-male sex.

After the serologic test was instituted, it was widely believed that with exclusion of high-risk donors and screening of all donations for antibodies to HIV, the blood supply was very safe. In 1988, however, John Ward and colleagues from the Centers for Disease Control (CDC) published a report in the *New England Journal of Medicine*[3] describing 13 people who were apparently infected with HIV from screened blood and had subsequently developed AIDS. Some risk of transmission was obviously still present.

Three strategies have been used to evaluate the residual risk from screened blood. The first is to followup the recipients, people who have been transfused with screened blood, to see whether or not they develop an HIV infection. That was the approach that we took at Johns Hopkins. The second approach has been to test the blood in the blood banks by a more sensitive technique such as DNA PCR (deoxyribonucleic acid polymerase chain reaction). This was done by Vyas and Busch in San Francisco. The third technique uses mathematical models to estimate the infectious window period prior to seroconversion and the probability that an infected donor would be in the window period.

A study using the first of these methods involved three hospitals: my own institution (Johns Hopkins in Baltimore) and St. Luke's Episcopal and Texas Methodist, both in Houston.[4] The study's short name, FACTS, stands for Frequency of Agents Communicable by Transfusion Study. The initial objective was to evaluate the effectiveness of HIV screening of the blood supply. Evaluating the risks of human T-lymphotropic virus (HTLV) I/II and hepatitis transmission by transfusion was added later.

The patients were adult cardiac surgery patients operated on in one of these three hospitals. Evaluation of transfusion-related infections in this group had several advantages. First, they were very heavily transfused. Second, they had a very low risk for HIV infection by any other means. Third, over 90

---

[3]Ward, JW, SD Holmberg, JR Allen, DL Cohn, SE Critchley, SH Kleinman, BA Lenes, O Ravenholt, JR Davis, MG Quinn, et al. (1988). Transmission of human immunodeficiency virus (HIV) by blood transfusions screened as negative for HIV antibody. *New England Journal of Medicine, 318(8):* 473–478.

[4]Nelson, KE, JG Donahue, A Muñoz, ND Cohen, PM Ness, A Teague, VA Stambolis, DH Yawn, B Callicott, H McAllister, et al. (1992). Transmission of retroviruses from seronegative donors by transfusion during cardiac surgery. A multicenter study of HIV-1 and HTLV-I/II infections. *Annals of Internal Medicine, 117(7):* 554–559.

percent were still alive 6 months after the surgery, and the follow-up was very good.

Blood samples were obtained prior to the operation. During the initial hospitalization, medical records were reviewed. A postoperative sample was obtained 6 to 8 months after surgery, along with a questionnaire that asked about high-risk behavior for HIV or hepatitis infection. Evidence of hepatitis or other signs of a transfusion-related illness were sought, and any history of additional postoperative transfusions was obtained. Roughly 12,000 people enrolled in the study, of whom almost 80 percent or 9,294 were transfused. Very importantly, in this study we also followed the remaining 2,200 people who underwent a cardiac surgical procedure, which normally requires a transfusion, but who were not transfused. They served as an important internal control, particularly for hepatitis, because they can be used to estimate background rates of hepatitis in hospitalized cardiac surgical patients.

A total of 120,000 units were transfused; on average, each transfused patient received 13 units. Among the recipients of these units, we found two people who seroconverted to HIV positive, i.e., 0.0017 percent, or a point estimate of 1 infection per 60,000 units transfused. Neither patient had risk behavior for HIV infection other than transfusion. All of the donors of the two seroconverters were located, and they included one who acknowledged male-to-male sexual relations, although he had denied it at the time he donated blood; this donor seroconverted after donating blood. We found another donor who seroconverted to HIV positive after donating blood given to the second HIV-positive cardiac case. Thus, we were fairly confident that both of these cases were transfusion acquired.

Screening of donors for HTLV I antibodies was instituted in 1988, while our study was still under way. Therefore, we were able to compare directly the impact of donor screening on postoperative HTLV incidence. There were a total of seven transfusion-associated HTLV I or II infections, only one of which occurred after donor screening was begun. This was a patient with HTLV II infection. The point estimate for HTLV II positivity was 1/67,000 units. Subsequent data have shown that the HTLV I screening test is not quite as sensitive in the detection of HTLV II infection. In fact, there is now some debate about the wisdom of adding HTLV II-specific antigens to the HTLV I screening in order to improve the sensitivity of the serological screening for HTLV II. However, HTLV II is not as clearly associated with human illness as HTLV I.

The second of the three approaches to estimating the risk of HIV transmission from HIV antibody-screened blood was taken by G.N. Vyas and colleagues at the Irwin Memorial Blood Center in San Francisco. They pooled blood samples from 50 donors and did cultures and a polymerase chain reaction test (PCR) in an attempt to detect the presence of HIV directly.[5] They identified one positive sample in the first pool, but none in 1,900 subsequent pools. Therefore, their estimate was 1 in 160,000 units (which is not statistically different from the 1/60,000 estimate of FACTS).

Another approach to estimating the risk was recently reported by Lyle Petersen and colleagues at the CDC.[6] They first identified repeat donors who had seroconverted. Then they did a look-back at outcomes for patients transfused with those donations. They found 561 repeat donors who had seroconverted and whose units had been transfused. Information was obtained on 182 recipients, of whom 36 had seroconverted to HIV positive since transfusion. When they modeled the interval between the last negative donation and the first positive donation to estimate when seroconversion might have occurred, the curve that best fit the data showed a median interdonation interval of 45 days for the donors whose antibody-screened blood led to seroconversion in recipients. Based upon this mathematical model, the group at CDC hypothesized that the median interval from the point at which a donor becomes infectious until the enzyme-linked immunosorbent assay (ELISA) for antibodies to HIV-1 and HIV-2 become positive was 45 days.

In a recent study published in *Transfusion*,[7] Busch et al. investigated whether current screening procedures have significantly shortened this seronegative window period. This study used donors who were PCR positive but antibody negative and who were subsequently found to have seroconverted, i.e., became positive on tests for the presence of antibodies to HIV. The interval from PCR positivity to antibody positivity could be estimated with these data. The PCR-positive sample was then tested with a number of more sensitive tests for the detection of HIV antibodies, antigens, or nucleic acid that are now available. This study showed that one-third to one-half of these seroconverters could be detected earlier with the current, more sensitive ELISAs: 80 percent were RNA (ribonucleic acid) PCR positive, and roughly 60 percent were p24 antigen-positive.

---

[5]Busch, MP, BE Eble, H Khayam-Bashi, et al. (1991). Evaluation of screened blood donations for human immunodeficiency virus type 1 infection by culture and DNA amplification of pooled cells. *New England Journal of Medicine, 325:* 2–5.

[6]Petersen, LR, GA Satten, R Dodd, M Busch, S Kleinman, A Grindon, B Lenes (1994). Duration of time from onset of human immunodeficiency virus type 1 infectiousness to development of detectable antibody. The HIV Seroconversion Study Group. *Transfusion, 34(4):* 283–289.

[7]Busch, MP, LL Lee, GA Satten, DR Henrard, H Farzadegan, KE Nelson, S Read, RY Dodd, LR Petersen (1995). Time course of detection of viral and serologic markers preceding human immunodeficiency virus type 1 seroconversion: Implications for screening of blood and tissue donors. *Transfusion, 35(2):* 91–97.

Taking the time to onset of infectiousness as marked by PCR positivity, the second-generation antibody assays (ELISA) reduced the seronegative window period by 6 days, the third generation assays reduced the window by about 19 days, and PCR and p24 antigen assays cut it even further. At present the seronegative window period is probably about 20 to 25 days or shorter. Because that is an average, some people will have longer windows and some will have some shorter, but there has been a substantial reduction in the window period with newer assays.

A study that is ongoing, the Retrovirus Epidemiology Donors Study (REDS), funded by the National Heart, Lung and Blood Institute, began in 1989 and is to continue until 1998. Its purpose is to monitor the safety of the nation's blood supply by studying donors who test positive, using a case control methodology with seronegative donors as controls. Five blood centers are involved in REDS, and so far the study has included 2.3 million donations from almost 586,000 multiple donors during a three-year period. Again, using data from the multiple donors that seroconvert, one can estimate the incidence and the length of the window period. If the HIV-1 incidence is multiplied by the length of the window period in repeat donors, one can estimate the rate of false-seronegative donations during the window.[8]

In a paper that Michael Busch presented at the National Institute of Health (NIH) Consensus Development Conference in January 1995, he reported 33 cases of HIV infection in repeat donors in 822,000 person years, for an overall incidence rate of 4 per 100,000 person years.[9] Using a window period estimate of 22 days yields an estimated risk of transfusion during the window period of 2.4 per million (1 in 416,000). The HIV prevalence rates in first-time donors are higher, which could also mean that HIV incidence may be higher among first-time donors, and therefore they are at higher risk of being in the window period. Despite this possible underestimation of the risk using this method, the estimate is probably fairly accurate.

We now have estimates of the risk of HIV infection from screened blood from four different studies. One was a follow-up of recipients in which the estimated risk was 1 in 60,000. A study with PCR estimated a risk of about 1 in 150,000. A mathematical model that was published in the *New England*

---

[8]Schreiber, GB, MP Busch, SH Kleinman, JJ Korelitz (1996). The risk of transfusion-transmitted viral infections. *New England Journal of Medicine, 334:* 1685–1690.

[9]Busch, MP (1995). Incidence of infectious disease markers in blood donors: Implications for residual risk of viral transmission by transfusion (abstract). NIH Consensus Development Conference on Infectious Disease Testing for Blood Transfusions, January 9–11, 1995, Bethesda, Maryland.

Journal of Medicine,[10] using all the Red Cross data for the 2 or 3 years after screening began, estimated a risk at 1 in 153,000. Finally, the mathematical model based on the Red Cross data estimates a risk of transfusion-transmitted HIV of 1 in 420,000 blood donors.[11]

The actual risk of HIV infection in HIV-seronegative donors is somewhat higher than the last figure, probably about 1 in 350,000, but other screening tests, namely the hepatitis B virus (HBV) core antibody test, the alanine aminotransferase (ALT) test, and the serologic test for syphilis, actually function as surrogate markers for HIV, eliminating some HIV-infected but antibody-negative donors because of positivity on these other screening tests. In fact, one of the reasons for the recent NIH Consensus Development Conference recommendation to retain the HBV core antibody test was for its value as a surrogate marker for HIV (as well as a direct marker for HBV infection). However, the HBV core antibody test was originally developed as a surrogate marker for hepatitis non-A, non-B.

Nearly every year since 1985 new tests and screening procedures have been introduced in an effort to reduce the risk of transfusion-transmitted infection from blood and blood products. More effective serologic screening, recruiting more repeat donors, screening rigorously by questionnaire, and confidential unit exclusion all have been used to combat the risk of disease transmission and have resulted in a four- or fivefold decrease in the prevalence of HIV infection in donors. Some people feel, and the REDS data would support this, that perhaps p24 antigen screening of the donors would further reduce the residual small risk of transfusion-transmitted HIV.

I would also like to describe some studies I have been involved with in a blood bank in the city of Chiang Mai, in northern Thailand, where the risk of infection from blood transfusion is very much higher than it is in the United States. In Thailand the rate of HIV-seropositive donors over the last six years has been about 3 to 4 percent. In this setting of a very high seroprevalence in blood donors, most of whom are neither male homosexuals nor intravenous drug users, the exclusion of these high-risk donors had much less impact than it has had in the United States. Therefore, it seemed reasonable to evaluate the effectiveness of screening donor blood for p24 antigen. In testing some 44,000 donors, we found 48 who were p24 antigen positive, 7 of whom did not have HIV-1 antibody and were neutralizable (and therefore were infected with HIV-

---

[10]Cumming, PD, EL Wallace, JB Schorr, RY Dodd (1989). Exposure of patients to human immunodeficiency virus through the transfusion of blood components that test antibody-negative. *New England Journal of Medicine, 321:* 941–946.

[11]Lackritz, EM, GA Satten, J Aberle-Grasse, et al. (1995). Estimated risk of transmission of the human immunodeficiency virus by screened blood in the United States. *New England Journal of Medicine, 333:* 1721–1725.

1 but in the seronegative window period). In a two-year period, p24 antigen screening detected 7 more infected donors that would have been missed by standard antibody screening tests.

In this study the ratio between antibody positivity (1519 donors) and antigen prevalence in antibody-negative donors (7 donors) was 1:217. If this ratio held true in the United States, where roughly 1 in 10,000 donors is antibody positive and there are about 13 million donors per year, we might exclude 6 additional HIV-infected donors with p24 antigen screening of all blood donations. The current estimate of the number of HIV-infected donors in the United States can be calculated from the risk data presented above. If the risk is 1 in 420,000 units and 13 million units per year are collected, then we might expect roughly 50 HIV infections per year. Reducing that number by 6 to 10 would constitute a 15 to 20 percent reduction. In Thailand the cost of p24 antigen testing is only a little over $4,000 for each transfusion infection prevented. The comparable figure in the United States would be somewhere in the $5 million to $10 million range to prevent one transfusion-transmitted HIV infection.

There is a second important virus that has been known to be a transfusion risk for some time. In the late 1970s and early 1980s, after the advent of screening of blood donors for HBV infection and after testing for infection with hepatitis A virus was introduced, it became clear that a large number of transfusion-transmitted hepatitis cases still occurred. This newly recognized type of hepatitis was called non-A, non-B hepatitis, and the search for the responsible virus began.

Several studies have examined whether testing donors for surrogate markers would prevent some cases of non-A, non-B hepatitis (now identified as being primarily due to infection with a third hepatitis virus, HCV).[12] Three studies showed roughly a twofold reduction in the risk of posttransfusion hepatitis associated with transfusion of blood tested and found to be negative

---

[12] Aach, RD, W Szmuness, JW Mosley, FB Hollinger, R Kahn, CE Stevens, VM Edwards, J Werch (1981). Serum alanine aminotransferase of donors in relation to the risk of non-A, non-B hepatitis in recipients: The transfusion-transmitted viruses study. *New England Journal of Medicine, 304:* 989–994. Stevens, CE, RD Aach, FB Hollinger, JW Mosley, W Szmuness, R Kahn, J Werch, VM Edwards, (1984). Hepatitis B virus antibody in blood donors and the occurrence of non-A, non-B hepatitis in transfusion recipients: An analysis of the transfusion-transmitted viruses study. *Annals of Internal Medicine, 101:* 733–738. Koziol, DC, PV Holland, DW Alling, JC Melpolder, RE Solomon, RH Purcell, LM Hudson, FJ Shoup, H. Krakaven, HJ Alter (1986). Antibody to hepatitis B core antigen as a paradoxical marker for non-A, non-B hepatitis agents in donated blood. *Annals of Internal Medicine, 104:* 488–495. Aynard, JP, C Janot, S Gayet, C Guillemin, P Canton, P Gardner, F Streiff (1986). Post-transfusion non-A, non-B hepatitis after cardiac surgery: Prospective analysis of donor blood anti-HBc antibody as a predictive indicator of the occurrence of non-A, non-B hepatitis in recipients. *Vox Sanguinis, 51:* 236–238.

for HBV core antibodies (compared to the rates when HBV core antibody positive blood had been transfused). Within a couple of years of these studies, blood banks began testing for antibodies to HBV core antigen and for alanine aminotransferase (ALT), in part as a result of the great public concern about blood safety associated with the AIDS epidemic.

The Johns Hopkins-Houston study of cardiac surgery patients, already described, was still in progress. Therefore, we were able to examine the efficacy of surrogate marker testing on the incidence of posttransfusion HCV infection as soon as the first-generation test for HCV became available. The study included three periods of donor screening: one soon after the start of HIV screening but before the start of surrogate marker (i.e., anti-HBV core and ALT) testing, which was begun in March 1985 and lasted until September 1986; a second period, between October 1986 and May 1990; and the third period, which began with the use of a specific test for donor antibodies to HCV in May 1990.

Our data indicate that the risk of HCV infection associated with transfusion was substantial prior to screening foe surrogate markers or HCV antibodies.[13] There is about an 18-fold difference in the rate of HCV infection attributable to transfusion: 366 cases occurred in 9,821 patients who were transfused but only 5 in the 2,400 who were not. The decline in transfusion-associated HCV infection with screening of donors for surrogate markers was significant regardless of which generation ELISA was used to test recipients, as was the much larger decrease after donor testing for anti-HCV antibody. About twice as many seroconverters were detected by the second generation ELISA, but there were also more indeterminate tests with the confirmatory radioimmunoblot assay (RIBA).[14] Testing these indeterminate samples by PCR and a third generation RIBA showed that only about a third of them were actually infected with HCV. The second-generation assay is now used to screen donors, so the best estimate of the current risk is about 3 per 10,000.

A recent paper by Blajchman and colleagues from Canada[15] reported a controlled study in which they assigned 4,500 patients to receive blood that either was or was not tested for surrogate markers (anti-HBV core antigen and

---

[13]Donahue, JG, A Muñoz, PM Ness, DE Brown, DH Yawn, HA McAlister, BA Reitz, KE Nelson (1992). The declining risk of post-transfusion hepatitis C virus infection. *New England Journal of Medicine, 327:* 369–373.

[14]Nelson, KE, F Ahmed, PM Ness, V Strumbolis, C Parniss, G Gosch, D Yawn, V McAlister (1993). Comparison of first and second generation ELISA screening tests in detecting HCV infections in transfused cardiac surgery patients. *Transfusion, 33(5):* 5116.

[15]Blajchman, MA, SB Bull, SV Feinman (1995). Post-transfusion hepatitis: Impact of non-A, non-B hepatitis surrogate tests. *Lancet, 345(8941):* 21–25.

ALT). Unlike the United States, Canada had not required surrogate marker screening on the basis of the data from the three studies cited above. However, while the study was in progress, anti-HCV testing was introduced throughout Canada. The results of this study generally confirmed the findings from our study. Prior to the institution of the specific test for HCV, roughly 20 seroconverters were seen per 1,000 units of untested blood transfused. Screening for surrogate markers reduced this rate to 5 per 1,000 units. After HCV testing was instituted there was still a small difference associated with surrogate marker screening of donors, but it was not significant. An important issue that blood banks are now facing is whether surrogate marker testing should be continued in the face of a sensitive and specific test for HCV. Most experts think that such testing is no longer justified by reduction of the risk of HCV. Indeed, in 1995 the NIH Consensus Development Conference advocated dropping ALT testing but continuing the use of anti-HBV core antigen screening because of its utility in reducing the risk of transfusion-transmitted HIV and HBV.

The risk of transmitting HBV by transfusion is a continuing concern to those working to improve the safety of the blood supply. In fact, HBV was the first viral infection for which donors were screened. Screening of donors for HBV infection began when the hepatitis B surface antigen (HBsAg) test was licensed in 1972. Nevertheless, there have been several case reports of people who have been infected with HBV despite screening for HBsAg. These HBV infections among persons receiving HBsAg screened blood could have occurred for several reasons. In an HBV-infectious donor the HBsAg test could be negative because HBsAg was present only at a level below the sensitivity of the assay, it was bound to antibody as an immune complex, or the HBV strain was a mutant virus without a surface antigen detectable by the current screening test.

The Hopkins-Houston cardiac surgery study allowed an estimate of the risk of transfusion-transmitted HBV and an assessment of the utility of other markers. To estimate the rate of transfusion-transmitted HBV, we screened transfused patients before and 6 months after their transfusion for antibodies to HBV core antigen. There was only about a twofold increase in the rate of incident HBV infections in the transfused patients compared to the incidence among those who were not transfused; the incidence of HBV infections among transfused patients was about tenfold lower per unit of blood than we found for HCV infections in the same study population. However, 39 patients seroconverted to HBV positivity after transfusion.

Interestingly, the method of donor screening had a significant effect on the rates of posttransfusion HBV infections in this population. HBV infection rates started at about 0.048 percent prior to surrogate marker screening and fell only to 0.039 percent with non-A, non-B surrogate marker testing (anti-HBV core antigen and ALT). After HCV testing was instituted, HBV seroconversion fell to a rate of 4 per 100,000 units transfused.[16]

These data suggest that HCV infection might be a surrogate for hepatitis B virus infections in donors. We studied this issue further by identifying donors to the Baltimore/Washington, D.C. Red Cross who tested positive for hepatitis C and examining their sera for other markers of HBV infection. Surprisingly, only 36 percent of these HCV-positive donors were without other markers. Many had anti-HBV core antibodies, elevated ALT or both, suggesting that the algorithm for testing now in use may actually prevent some infections from viruses other than their target. Similarly, ALT testing may have improved the safety with regard to transmission of HBV.

James Moseley did another analysis that supports our data. He found 15 recipients among patients enrolled in the Transfusion Transmitted Viruses Study of the 1970s[17] who seroconverted to HBV positive when transfused with hepatitis B surface antigen-negative blood. Moseley then tested the original samples from these patients with current tests for hepatitis B surface antigen, HBV core antibody, and HBV-DNA PCR. Six of the 15 were core antibody positive. These data suggest that if we had tested donors for HBV core antibody in the middle and late 1970s, we might have prevented some transfusion-related HBV infections even though these donors had been found negative for hepatitis B surface antigen.

The incidence of infection with HIV, HTLV, HCV, and HBV has very recently been determined for the 586,507 repeat donors in REDS. These data, together with the estimated duration of the seronegative window periods for these infections, were used to estimate the risk of transmission by transfusion between 1991 and 1993.[18] This study estimated the residual risks of transmission of these viruses from transfusion of screened blood as 1 in 493,000 donor units for HIV, 1 in 641,000 donor units for HTLV, 1 in 103,000 donor units for HCV, and 1 in 63,000 donor units for HBV.

Another disease that has assumed increased importance as a transfusion-transmitted infection is Chagas' disease, or *Trypanosoma cruzi* infections. In much of South and Central America there are focal areas where people are

---

[16] Nelson, KE (1995). The risk of the transmission of retroviruses, hepatitis C virus and hepatitis B virus according to the methods of donor screening (abstract). NIH Consensus Development Conference on Infectious Disease Testing for Blood Transfusions, January 9–11, 1995, Bethesda, Maryland.

[17] Mosley, JW, CE Stevens, RD Aach, FB Halligen, LT Mimmus, LR Solomon, CH Barbasn, GJ Nemo (1995). Donor screening for antibody to hepatitis B core antigen and hepatitis B virus infection in transfusion to recipients. *Transfusion, 35:* 5–12.

[18] Schreiber, GB, MP Busch, SH Kleinman, JJ Korelitz (1996). The risk of transfusion-transmitted viral infections. *New England Journal of Medicine, 334:* 1685–1690.

carriers of *T. cruzi* and can transmit the infection by blood transfusion. Four cases have now been reported in the United States and Canada. As a result, Roger Dodd and his group at the Red Cross[19] began a study in two blood banks, in Los Angeles and Miami, that were considered to have a donor population who might be at high risk for infection with *T. cruzi*. They screened all donors by questionnaire to ascertain whether they had ever resided for more than 4 weeks in an area where Chagas disease is endemic. Among 91,216 donors, 6,302 said yes, and their blood was tested for *T. cruzi*. Twenty-three were positive on an initial enzyme immunoassay, and 10 of them were confirmed to be positive by radioimmunoprecipitation assay.

I would like to conclude by calling your attention to an important risk that has not, in my opinion, been adequately addressed, namely transfusion-transmitted bacterial infections.[20] Many papers in the literature have reported on the transmission of *Yersinia enterocolitica* infection by transfusion from apparently healthy blood donors. *Y. enterocolitica* is one of a number of organisms that can cause asymptomatic bacteremia in donors and survive and replicate in the cold temperatures at which blood is stored. More recently there has been some focus on the risks associated with the transfusion of platelets, which must be stored at room temperature to preserve their function. In one study that evaluated 35,000 platelet transfusions, 37, or about 1 in 1000, were associated with febrile episodes. Ten of these episodes were shown to be bacteremic. The risk of bacteremia per unit of platelets transfused was 1 in 2,000.

Contamination of platelets by staphylococcal and other organisms that are normal skin flora during the donation process is not uncommon. In the four or five days that the platelets may be stored at room temperature, there may be enough bacterial growth for the recipient to develop a significant infection after transfusion of these platelets even if visual inspection at the time of use uncovers no sign of bacterial growth.

In order to evaluate a procedure to reduce this risk, Yomtovian and her colleagues at the Cleveland Clinic[21] have cultured or done Gram stains in order to identify bacterial contamination of platelets. They then deferred transfusion of platelets found to be positive and found a significant decrease

---

[19]Dodd, RY (1995). Preventing transfusion-transmitted Chagas disease: the American Red Cross approach (abstract). NIH Consensus Development Conference on Infectious Disease Testing for Blood Transfusions, January 9–11, 1995, Bethesda, Maryland.

[20]Blajchman, MA (1994). Transfusion-associated bacterial sepsis: The phoenix rises yet again. *Transfusion, 34:* 940–942.

[21]Yomtovian, R, HM Lazarus, LT Goodnough, NV Hirschler, AM Morrissey, MR Jacobs (1993). A prospective microbiologic surveillance program to detect and prevent the transfusion of bacterially contaminated platelets. *Transfusion, 33:* 902–909.

in the rate of bacteremia in recipients of the culture- and Gram stain-negative platelets. However, another study using Gram status or culture to identify units of platelets at high risk of causing bacterial sepsis concluded that these techniques were poor sreening methods because of their inadequte sensitivity and specificity.[22] Clearly, more research needs to be done in order to develop sensitive, specific, and practical methods for reducing the risks of the transfusion transmission of bacterial infections, especially those associated with platelet transfusion.

The occurrence of transfusion-transmitted HIV and a better understanding of the high frequency of chronic hepatitis C virus infections have obviously led to a greater appreciation of the potential importance of transfusion acquired infections. What will the future bring? It seems inevitable that we will discover new pathogens that are transmissible by the transfusion of blood products. Indeed, researchers have recently identified and sequenced a new flavivirus that is carried in the blood of approximately 1 percent of blood donors and is transmittable by transfusion.[23] Although it has been named hepatitis G virus (HGV), preliminary clinical data suggest that individuals who have acquired HGV infections do not seem to develop chronic hepatitis despite chronic infection with HGV.[24]

The strains of HIV-1 that have caused the worldwide pandemic of AIDS have been designated as group M viruses. Another group of HIV-1 viruses have been identified that cause AIDS but show extensive genetic divergence from group M strains.[25] These HIV-1 viruses have been designated group O viruses. The antibody response elicited by these group O strains is not

---

[22] Barrett, BB, JW Anderson, KC Anderson (1993). Strategies for the avoidance of bacterial contamination of blood components. *Transfusion, 33:* 228–234.

[23] Simons, JN, TP Leavy, GJ Dawson, TJ Pilot-Matis, AS Muerhoff, GG Schlauder, SM Desai, IK Mushahwar (1995). Isolation of novel virus-like sequences associated with human hepatitis. *Nature Medicine 1:* 564–569. Linnen, J, J Wages Jr, ZY Zhang-Keck, KE Fry, HZ Krawczynski, H Alter, E Koonin, M Gallagher, M Alter, S Hadzlyannis (1996). Molecular cloning and disease association of hepatitis G virus: A transfusion-transmissible agent. *Science, 271:* 505–508. Simons, JN, TJ Pilot-Matis, TP Leavy, GJ Dawson, SM Desai, GG Schlauder, AS Muerhoff, JC Erker, SJ Buijk, ML Chalmers (1995). Identification of two flavivirus-like genomes in the GB hepatitis agent. *Proceedings of the National Academy of Sciences USA, 92:* 3401–3405.

[24] Alter, HJ, Y Nakatsuji, JW-K Shih, J Melpolder, K Kiyosawa, J Wages, J Kim (1996). Tranfusion-associated hepatitis G virus infection (abstract 120). Paper presented at the IX Triennial International Symposium on Viral Hepatitis and Liver Diseases, Rome, Italy, April 21–25. Alter, M, M Gallagher, T Morris, C Moyer, K Krawczyaski, Y Khadyakow, H Fields, J Kim, A Margolis (1996). Epidemiology of non A-non E hepatitis (abstract 119). Paper presented at the IX Triennial International Symposium on Viral Hepatitis and Liver Diseases, Rome, Italy, April 21–25.

[25] Gurtler, LG, PH Hauser, J Eberle (1994). A new subtype of human immunodeficiency virus type 1 (MVP-5180) from Cameroon. *Journal of Virology, 68:* 1581–1585.

consistently detected by currently licensed ELISA kits.[26] Most persons infected with group O viruses have been from West and Central Africa, especially Cameroon, Gabon, Nigeria, Niger, Senegal and Togo. However, one patient from Los Angeles and a French national have been found to be infected with HIV-1 group O strains.[27] Several companies are developing ELISA screening tests that will detect both group O and group M strains of HIV-1, but none of these assays are currently licensed by FDA. These case suggest that there will be a continuing need for rapid development, evaluation, and licensure of new screening tests in order to maintain the safety of the blood supply.

---

[26]Loussert-Ajaka, I, TD Ly, ML Chaix (1994). HIV-1/HIV-2 seronegativity in HIV-1 subtype O infected patients. *Lancet, 344:* 1333–1334.

[27]Centers for Disease Control and Prevention (1996). Identification of HIV-1 group O infection—1996. *Morbidity and Mortality Weekly Report, 45:* 561–565.

Viral Inactivation of Blood Products: A General Overview

Bernard Horowitz

Over the past decade, blood banking and blood processing procedures and the practice of transfusion medicine have changed substantially. Today, we are more aware of the dangers of blood transfusion and of steps to reduce if not eliminate these dangers. Blood donors are examined and questioned more closely than ever before in an attempt to eliminate donors who are more likely to harbor an infectious blood-borne virus. Every donation is tested by new and more sensitive blood tests, and in some cases blood screening tests are introduced even before their benefit is established. Donor histories and test results have been computerized, and the error-prone manual transcription of critical information is being eliminated. Manufactured blood products are more highly purified than ever before, and purification procedures have been modified to more consistently reduce viral load.

Virus inactivation technology is in widespread use in the preparation of coagulation factor concentrates, and validated virus inactivation methods are beginning to be applied to all blood protein solutions including immune globulins and fresh frozen plasma (FFP). One could not fathom introduction of a new blood protein product today if it was not virally inactivated.

With respect to viral safety, the data are clear: the only way to achieve absolute safety is through viral inactivation, and numerous advantages accrue on adoption of virus inactivation processes. The window period of seronegativity will no longer be of concern, errors in testing or the inadvertent release of a blood unit that tests positive will no longer result in viral transmission, new viruses or new viral serotypes will be eliminated even before their presence is recognized, and tests for rare viruses need not be deployed.

Nowhere can the value of virus inactivation be illustrated better than in the preparation of coagulation factor concentrates. Antihemophilic factor (AHF) concentrate and prothrombin complex concentrate manufactured without viral inactivation transmitted human immunodeficiency virus (HIV), hepatitis

B virus (HBV), and hepatitis C virus (HCV) at high frequency.[28] As late as 1985, essentially every vial of these concentrates was contaminated by HCV. With the advent of viral inactivation, HIV transmission was virtually eliminated. For example, in the United States not a single documented case of HIV transmission has been associated with concentrate infusion since 1987. In fact, solvent/detergent- (S/D-) treated products are used in the preparation of approximately two-thirds of the world's plasma-derived coagulation factor concentrates, and more than 7 million doses have been infused without a single documented case of HIV, HBV, or HCV transmission (see Table 1).

TABLE 1 S/D-Treated Product Usage: 1985–March 1994

Product	Units	Doses (approx.)
Factor VII	1.9 MU	1,900
Factor VIIa	2.6 MU	2,600
Factor VIII	6,085 MU	6,085,000
Factor IX	353 MU	353,000
Prothrombin complex	113 MU	105,667
Fibrin glue	325,930 ml	65,186
Fibrinogen	93,300 g	23,300
IMIG & IVIG	1,266,245 g	253,249
MAb IgM	2,697 vials	2,697
Anti-D IgG	83,702 vials	83,702
Plasma	789,479 units	197,400
Sum		7,173,701

SOURCE: Horowitz, B, AM Prince, MS Horowitz, C Watklevicz (1993). Viral safety of solvent-detergent treated blood products. In Brown F (ed), Virological Safety Aspects of Plasma Derivatives, Developments in Biological Standardization, 81: 147–161; updated with information on file.

The commonly employed viral elimination procedures are:

- heat (pasteurization, dry heat, vapor),
- solvent/detergent,
- beta-propiolactone/ultraviolet light,
- acid,

---

[28] Horowitz, B, MPJ Piet (1986). Transmission of viral diseases by plasma protein fractions. *Plasma Therapy Transfusion Technology*, 7: 503–513.

- sodium thiocyanate,
- filtration,
- extensive purification, and
- combinations.

Each has distinctive features. S/D acts by disrupting the viral lipid envelope, and a 12-year history of safety with respect to enveloped viruses supports its use. Virus kill is rapid (≤ 1 hour) and complete. Because action is directed toward lipids, nonenveloped viruses and proteins (except for lipoproteins) are unaffected, and S/D can be applied equally and predictably with a high rate of recovery to complex mixtures such as plasma and to highly purified protein solutions. Safety with respect to HBV, HCV, and HIV is supported by 13 independently run clinical trials.

Methods of thermal inactivation are advantageous in that all classes of virus are potentially susceptible, although nonenveloped viruses tend to be heat stable. Because thermal inactivation methods are not inherently specific, means of stabilizing proteins while achieving excellent virus inactivation had to be identified. With pasteurization, proteins are stabilized by addition of high concentrations of low-molecular-weight solutes, especially sugars and amino acids. Although viruses are also stabilized, relatively good discrimination can be achieved, although at some cost in protein recovery. Using the duck HBV as a model, S/D treatment is more effective than pasteurization at killing HBV.[29] Additionally, many nonenveloped viruses are also heat resistant.

With dry heat, proteins are stabilized by reducing the moisture content, and process recovery can be high. A particular advantage of the dry heat method is that it can be performed on product in the final container, eliminating the possibility of posttreatment recontamination. With all other methods, recontamination is prevented by separating pre- and postvirus inactivation areas, equipment, and personnel. Nonetheless, despite these differences, each method has eliminated HIV transmission by pooled plasma products, and HBV and HCV transmission has either been eliminated or greatly reduced.[30]

More recently, the apparent transmission of hepatitis A virus (HAV) by an ion-exchange-purified, S/D-treated AHF concentrate in several European countries raised concerns about nonenveloped viruses, first because they are

---

[29]Long, Z, C-S Sun, EM White, B Horowitz, AF Sito (1993). Hepatitis B viral clearance studies using duck virus model. In Brown F (ed): Virological Safety Aspects of Plasma Derivatives. *Developments in Biological Standardization, 81:* 163–168.

[30]Horowitz, B (1991). Inactivation of viruses found with plasma proteins. In Goldstein, J (ed.), *Biotechnology of Blood.* Boston: Butterworth-Heinemann.

not inactivated by S/D treatment and second because they tend to be heat stable. Viruses in this class include HAV and parvovirus B19. Consequently, manufacturers are examining newer viral elimination procedures in combination with established virucidal procedures.

The advantage of combining methods that act by independent mechanisms is that both a broader spectrum and a higher quantity of viruses can be eliminated. As examples, antibody affinity purification validated as a virus removal method has been combined with either S/D or heat treatment; some products are now treated by both S/D and heat; other products have been processed through virus-removing filters that have been developed recently and added to existing processes. New methods of viral inactivation under exploration include the use of chaotropes such as sodium thiocyanate, short-wavelength ultraviolet light in the presence of antioxidants, microwave heating, extraction with supercritical fluids, and iodine. Given the extensive history of safety with respect to the principal viruses of concern achieved by currently employed methods, it seems likely that these techniques will supplement rather than replace existing processes. As an example, research at the New York Blood Center has shown that combining S/D with ultraviolet C irradiation kills a wide variety of viruses including HBV, HCV, HIV, HAV, and parvovirus (Table 2).

TABLE 2 Viral Elimination by Combination of S/D and Ultraviolet C Light (UVC)[a]

Virus	Viral Elimination ($\log_{10}$)		
	SD	UVC	Sum
VSV	>6.5	4.4	>10.9
Sindbis	>6.3	>6.0	>12.3
HBV	>6.0	na	>6.0
HCV	>5.0	na	>5.0
HIV	>6.2	>5.6	>11.8
EMC	0	>5.6	>5.6
HAV	0[b]	>5.3	>5.3
Parvovirus	0	>5.0	>5.0

[a] Abbreviations: VSV, vesicular stomatitus virus; EMC, encephalomypcarditis virus; na, not available
[b] S/D enhances immune neutralization

Thus, despite being prepared from plasma pools, today's coagulation factor concentrates have proven to be safe from transmission of HBV, HCV, and HIV. Virally inactivated concentrates are now safer than the individual units from which they were derived. Success with the sterilization of coagulation factor concentrates encourages research into the sterilization of blood components, i.e., FFP, red blood cell concentrates (RBCCs) and platelet concentrates.

Before addressing the viral inactivation of blood components, we must ask if individual units of blood are already safe enough. It is my belief that the goal should be to reduce viral risk to 1 per 1 million or less, and that this goal can only be achieved through virus inactivation.

Transfusion Plasma. Our experience with S/D encouraged us to develop S/D-treated plasma (SD-plasma) as a substitute for fresh frozen plasma (FFP). Briefly, units of FFP are combined, thawed, and treated with 1% tri(n-butyl)phosphate (TNBP) and 1% Triton X-100 at 30°C for four hours, the reagents removed by hydrophobic chromatography. The final product is then sterile filtered, frozen, and optionally, lyophilized. Viral inactivation has been extensively validated. Under these conditions of S/D treatment, the rate of VSV and Sindbis virus killing exceeds that observed with AHF concentrates, treated either with TNBP-cholate or TNBP-Tween. We have also shown that $\geq 10^6$ infectious doses (ID_{50}) of HBV, $\geq 10^5$ ID_{50} of HCV, and $\geq 10^{7.2}$ ID_{50} of HIV are killed and that $\geq 10^{4.5}$ ID_{50} of HAV are neutralized. Because of pooling, a dose of SD-plasma consistently has 30 times more anti-HAV antibody than a dose of intramuscular immune globulin, known to prevent the spread of HAV, and has approximately the same quantity of antiparvovirus antibody as a dose of intravenous immune globulin, reported to be effective in the therapy of parvovirus infections. The coagulation factor content resembles that of the start pool and is more consistent than that found in individual donor units. There is no evidence that coagulation factors are activated, and the level of other proteins is normal. Toxicology studies indicate that the tiny amounts of TNBP and Triton X-100 that remain are safe.

SD-plasma has been extensively evaluated in the United States and Europe.[31] In the United States, more than 20 clinical study sites took part. In our own studies, 93 patients were treated on 504 occasions with 1,334 units of SD-Plasma. This included the successful treatment of 37 surgical episodes and 75 bleeding episodes in patients who were congenitally coagulation factor deficient and 9 successful uses to reverse warfarin therapy in advance of surgery. In patients with chronic or acute thrombotic thrombocytopenic purpura, SD-plasma was just as good as FFP in stimulating an increase in platelet count. Formal viral safety studies indicate that virus has not been

---

[31]Pehta, JC (1994). Clinical studies with solvent detergent-treated plasma. *Transfusion Medicine Audio Updates.*

transmitted, and this conclusion is supported by published studies[32] and the more than 1 million units infused in Europe to date.

Blood Cell Concentrates. Sterilization of cellular products is more difficult than virus inactivation of blood protein products, because blood cells are more complex and fragile than proteins, and multiple viral forms are present, including cell-free virus, virus that is adherent to cell membranes, actively replicating virus, and latently infected cells. Nonetheless, because erythrocytes and platelets do not replicate, methods that modify membranes or nucleic acid may prove useful.

Red Blood Cell Concentrates. Numerous methods have been investigated, including the use of beta-propiolactone, nitrogen mustards, aryl diol epoxides, ozone, and halogenated oxidizing agents, but the best results described thus far employ photodynamically active sensitizers and visible light. Early work by Matthews and coworkers[33] showed good virus kill with hematoporphyrin derivative. We have shown that by substituting phthalocyanine, which absorbs light where hemoglobin does not, virus kill is greatly improved.[34]

Phthalocyanines and other dyes, like methylene blue or sapphyrins, activate oxygen to its reactive forms. With phthalocyanine treatment of red cell concentrates, we have begun to analyze the complex reaction pathways through the addition of quenchers of reactive oxygen species. Some compounds like mannitol and glutathione will quench oxygen radicals, while other compounds like tryptophan and sodium azide principally quench singlet oxygen. Using this approach we have shown that virus kill is not mediated by oxygen radicals but is mediated by singlet oxygen. This finding has practical importance because we can enhance reaction specificity by including quenchers of radicals at the time of light exposure.

Platelet Concentrates. Photodynamically active compounds such as those under evaluation in the treatment of RBCCs reduce platelet aggregation response to collagen and to other agonists, but encouraging results have been

---

[32]Inbal, A, O Epstein, D Blickstein, et al. (1993). Evaluation of solvent/detergent treated plasma in management of patients with hereditary and acquired coagulation disorders. *Blood Coagulation and Fibrinolysis, 4:* 599–604.

[33]Matthews, JL, JT Newman, F Sogandares-Bernal, et al. (1988). Photodynamic therapy of viral contaminants with the potential for blood banking applications. *Transfusion, 28:* 81–88.

[34]Horowitz, B, B Williams, S Rywkin, et al. (1991). Inactivation of viruses in blood with aluminum phthalocyanine derivatives. *Transfusion, 31:* 102–108.

obtained with psoralen derivatives. Psoralens are naturally occurring furocoumarins found in many foods, and they have been used therapeutically since antiquity. The principal reaction of psoralens on exposure to long-wavelength ultraviolet light is the cross-linking of nucleic acids. The initial report on the treatment of platelets with psoralens came from Corash's laboratory.[35] Treatment of an oxygen depleted platelet concentrate with 8'-methoxypsoralen and UVA irradiation was shown to inactivate ≥ 6.7 $\log_{10}$ CFU of *Escherichia coli*, ≥ 6.9 $\log_{10}$ CFU of *Staphylococcus aureus*, ≥ 7.3 $\log_{10}$ PFU of phage fd, 2.5 $\log_{10}$ PFU of phage R17, and 5.1 $\log_{10}$ PFU of feline leukemia virus. When treatment was under deoxygenated conditions, platelet morphology, process recovery, and response to the aggregation agent A23187 were comparable to thopse of untreated controls. If not first deoxygenated, aggregation response was adversely affected. We have overcome the deoxygenation requirement by adding quenchers of active oxygen species.[36] Additionally, new synthetic psoralens with increased reactivity with nucleic acids are being developed and may serve to enhance reaction specificity further.

In conclusion, blood and blood products have never been safer. However, the public's continuing concern about the safety of the blood supply from viruses, and the differential safety profile between blood and other pharmaceuticals demand that we continually improve. The achievements of the past are laudable. Nonetheless, safety from viruses falls well short of a standard of less than one transmission per 1 million units transfused, a realistic goal that we believe the transfusion community should adopt. For single-donor blood products, improved screening systems may achieve this goal; however, screening systems alone will never eliminate the window of seronegativity, and screening tests cannot anticipate new viruses or viral serotypes. Pooled blood products that have been virally inactivated meet this standard for most viruses, and use of a second viral elimination procedure that complements the first one will further ensure the safety of these products. Incorporation of viral inactivation procedures into the manufacture of all blood products, including blood cell concentrates, overcomes the weaknesses of screening procedures, and the further development of virus inactivation methodologies should continue to be encouraged.

---

[35]Lin, L, GP Wiesehahn, PA Morel, L Corash (1989). Use of 8-methoxypsoralen and long wave-length ultraviolet radiation for decontamination of platelet concentrates. *Blood, 74:* 517–525.

[36]Margolis-Nunno, H, R Robinson, E Ben-Hur, B Horowitz (1994). Quencher enhanced specificity of psoralen photosensitized virus inactivation in platelet concentrates. *Transfusion, 34:* 802–810.

II

Guarding the Blood Supply

The Retrovirus Epidemiology Donor Study: Rationale and Methods

Thomas F. Zuck

I am going to briefly outline the rationale and methods of the Retrovirus Epidemiology Donor Study (REDS). I am going to provide no data except to look at the enormity of the database that has been accumulated.

A request for proposals (RFP) was published in 1988 by the National Heart, Lung and Blood Institute (NHLBI), because of the unknown infectious risk of transfusion, concern about HIV variants, the need to understand human T-lymphotropic virus (HTLV) infection, a need to create repositories to examine emerging infectious agents, and a need to evaluate emerging technologies to detect these agents. The study will run from 1989 to 1998, and it is likely that it will be extended beyond then. The purpose is to monitor the safety of the nation's blood supply through studies of the epidemiology of known agents, essentially retroviruses, among volunteer blood donors.

What I am going to share with you today has recently been published in *Transfusion*.[37] Blood centers were selected on the basis of the quality of their proposals. There are four high-risk centers and one low-risk center, risk being defined as areas having a high background prevalence of AIDS. The REDS high-risk participants are the Red Cross Greater Chesapeake and Potomac, the Red Cross Southern Michigan, the Red Cross Southern California, and Irwin Memorial Blood Center. Oklahoma was considered to be low risk. The coordinating data center was Westat, Inc. The scope of the study is $40 million over the course of 5 years, and it is considered the most complicated study that NHLBI has ever launched.

The structure is governed by a steering committee that has two investigators from each of the participating centers and the committee is chaired by an independent center director, who happens to be me. Subcommittees of this steering committee developed the proposals and protocols that we have been following over the course of the study. We have a continuing and an ongoing close relationship with the Centers for Disease Control and Prevention (CDC).

---

[37]Zuck, TF, RA Thompson, GB Schreiber, RO Gilcher, et al. (1995). The retrovirus epidemiology donor study (REDS): Rationale and methods. *Transfusion, 35:* 944–951.

There are five major REDS components:

- monitoring donors,
- creating a general repository,
- creating special repositories,
- studying a cohort of people infected with HTLV, and
- surveying donors concerning the prevalence of certain behavioral and attitudinal issues.

Three substudies are pursuing these five objectives:

- establishing and maintaining a serum and cell repository,
- following the cohort of HTLV-infected donors and patients, and
- conducting the mail surveys directly.

There are three REDS repositories:

- the General Serum Repository,
- the General Leukocyte and Plasma Repository (GLPR), and
- a Special Repository.

Serum taken from donors routinely is selected at random based on a complicated sampling methodology devised by the statisticians at Westat. Samples in the special repositories are: donations that are repeatedly reactive for HTLV, but for which confirmatory testing is unclear; donations from sex partners of HTLV-positive subjects and their controls; donations that were repeatably reactive for HIV-1 but which produced indeterminate Western blots; donations that were repeatably reactive for HIV-2 but HIV-1 negative; and donations that were repeatably reactive for HIV but of unclear etiology.

The HTLV cohort study uses a case-control methodology to investigate HTLV risk and transmission factors and to define the natural history of HTLV infection. Other than some studies in Kyushu, Japan, we know little about the natural history of HTLV infection. One of its outcomes, T-cell leukemia, is so infrequent that it is difficult to estimate how often it occurs once an infection has been identified.

There were also few data on symptoms related to HTLV-associated myelopathy and tropical spastic paraparesis short of those two diseases themselves. They are actually identical conditions but defined in different parts of the world by different names. We were essentially searching for unexpected clinical outcomes, because in 1988, when this study was designed, the literature was unclear on the clinical outcomes of this infection.

The donor mail surveys were done in waves. The survey subjects were selected by sophisticated statistical techniques that randomized the selection of survey recipients. The resulting sample was enriched with donors from certain types of populations that we knew had high infection rates. The idea was to ascertain risk behaviors of the donors. The survey was stratified by several variables: center, race, age, sex, zip code, birth year, etc., trying to focus again on those people among the donor population who were more likely to engage in high-risk behaviors. This is randomized in a biased way in terms of enriching it for younger people. We mailed out about 64,000 questionnaires; the response rate was about 70 percent.

The most important outcome is the extensive databases that are available for use today. We have demographic information from the donors of 4.9 million donations. The General Serum Repository contains 500,000 samples stored in multiple vials which are now the property of NHLBI.

The GLPR has both leukocytes and plasma so that we can look at any kind of virus that may be only intracellular, such as HTLV, in which the genome is not free in the plasma. We have 546 HTLV-infected donors and patients who have been enrolled and who are being followed longitudinally for the presence or emergence of symptoms. The information in this database is immense and enormously valuable. To date, the surveys have found that more risky behavior is being encountered than predicted: up to 1 percent of people report prior drug use, sexual activity with a previous drug abuser, etc.

The extensive data also permit incidence calculations. One of the difficulties we have had over the years is dealing with prevalence. We know what our current rate of infection in the donor base is, but in the past we could not look at incident infections, that is, in how many people per year does it occur? Those calculations are now being made. They contribute to the decision making regarding HIV antigen testing in a negative way. They show that antigen testing is probably not of great public health value.

We have established an orderly process to access the database. An application is sent to the REDS Publication Committee, which looks at the request to see whether we want to provide a series of samples or process a request for data or data analysis. The committee then decides whether to recommend to NHLBI that the database or the samples be accessed for the requested purpose. NHLBI can veto the use of data or samples. This is particularly important for samples because once you have thawed them and then refrozen them, the test results gained from those thawed and refrozen samples have less credibility with certain kinds of testing technology. Thus NHLBI must carefully guard the repositories.

The contributions of REDS to date have been important, and I have outlined just a few here that are by no means all inclusive. We were also involved with a team dealing with the idiopathic CD4 lymphocytopenia (ICL) crisis. Within days of the report of ICL, REDS formed a task force with CDC.

CDC had a meeting that included two Nobel laureates within 3 or 4 weeks of the announcement in Amsterdam. We used the laboratory facilities of REDS to work with the technology for CD4 counting. There were some recommendations from the panel convened at CDC that perhaps we ought to screen for CD4 counts. We quickly mobilized several REDS labs. We found that the technology was not available to do it practically with reliable results. It turned out that the data from people with ICL, so-called people with "AIDS without virus," were merely outliers in the normal variation of T-cells counted in blood donors, although it took us a while to discover that. REDS was at the center of that, with incredible cooperation from the CDC.

REDS also developed consensus conference data that were presented both at an NIH Consensus Development Conference and at the Blood Products Advisory Committee. These involved incidence data and window period estimates for viral diseases and how much we would close the window by antigen testing and whether there would be a magnet effect. REDS will continue to make general contributions to the risk literature. We are still probably the largest database of donors that can be accessed quickly with a great deal of accuracy.

The Institute of Medicine report on *HIV and the Blood Supply* recommended continuing monitoring for risks in the blood supply. REDS is a very comprehensive database, and, importantly, can yield incidence data, and the use of incidence data is really the most reliable way to make decisions on what is happening. We can continue to track elements specified in the RFP which are the data elements that I have outlined. Most importantly, as with ICL and the lessons with ICL, we were able to respond within days because we had the five centers in place. We had Westat crunching the numbers. We were able to respond in a way that no one else can because of the magnitude of the database that we have to deal with.

One of the things that we might want to consider is not maintaining the current level of funding, but using a reduced level of funding to keep the REDS mechanism in place for the future so that we can respond and answer queries when we need to. It took us 18 months to set up this system. It was extremely difficult and it is extremely complicated, but it is in place now. It is on autopilot. It would be a pity if we lost the opportunity to have continuous surveillance and answer queries about unknown agents, new testing technologies, and the like.

Demographic and Serologic Characteristics of Volunteer Blood Donors[38]

James J. Korelitz

I would like to provide a brief overview of the demographic profile of blood donors in the Retrovirus Epidemiology Donor Study (REDS) as well as the prevalence of infectious markers that has been observed. I would then like to share with you the attempts to estimate the incidence of infectious disease markers, how incidence differs from prevalence, and how the incidence rate can be used in conjunction with estimates of periods of true positivity but seronegativity (window periods) to assess the risk of an infectious unit entering the blood supply.

In addition to standard questions, such as those regarding gender and age, REDS collects information on additional donor demographics such as race, ethnicity, education, country of birth, and transfusion history. The standard battery of serologic tests is performed on all donations including tests for retroviruses and hepatitis viruses. A key feature of REDS worth emphasizing is that a unique donor identifier is created so that donations from the same donor can be linked for further analyses such as the incidence analysis, as well as with other components of REDS.

What are the demographic characteristics of blood donors? Based on approximately 2,000,000 donations (excluding autologous) collected during 1991 and 1992, we found that

- slightly more donations are from males than from females,
- more than 70 percent of donations are from the 20–49 age group, with about 10 percent from those under 20 and about 20 percent from those 50 and older,
- over 80 percent of donations come from white, non-hispanic donors, and

---

[38]Talk presented at Forum on Blood Safety and Blood Availability, July 12–13, 1994. An updated analysis is given in Schreiber, GB, MP Busch, SH Kleinman, JJ Korelitz (1996). The risk of transfusion-transmitted viral infections. *New England Journal of Medicine, 334:* 1685–1690.

- donors are generally well-educated, 70 percent having some college experience and almost 90 percent being high school graduates.

An important factor that will come up when we talk about incidence is the fact that 79 percent of our donations are from repeat donors and 21 percent are from first-time donors. It has been generally recognized that first-time donors have a higher prevalence of infectious disease markers compared with repeat donors.

With that demographic profile in mind, what kind of prevalence values are we observing? During 1991 and 1992, the prevalence of human immunodeficiency virus (HIV) and human T-lymphotropic virus (HTLV) were each about 1 per 10,000 donations. For hepatitis C virus (HCV), based on 19 months of data corresponding to when the supplemental HCV test was implemented at the blood centers, the prevalence was about 22 per 10,000. Prevalence gives us an idea of how many people are currently infected, or positive, for an infectious disease marker. It has obvious importance, especially from a broad public health perspective, for estimating the current magnitude of a health problem.

However, prevalence does not provide us with any indication of when the infection occurred, and the timing of an infection is critical in the blood donor setting. After all, people who were infected long ago will show up as prevalent cases, but their donations will test positive and be excluded from the blood supply. A more important question relates to the rate at which negative donors are becoming positive, or seroconverting. People who have seroconverted will test positive, and their donations will be excluded, but people who are seroconverting may be in the window period where their donations are infectious but not detected by current tests.

The definition of an incident case is fairly straightforward: it is when a donor who previously gave a negative donation shows up and gives a positive one. Remember that with REDS we have a linking donor identification number, so these donors can be identified. The incidence rate is then calculated as the number of incident cases divided by the total person-time observed.

Let me give a brief example to explain person-time. Suppose person A gives two seronegative donations 18 months apart, and person B gives two seronegative donations 6 month apart. Neither one is an incident case, so we could say the incidence rate is 0 out of 2 donors. This method treats each donor equally. However, we would like to incorporate the fact that donor A was observed to remain seronegative for a longer time period than donor B. Likewise, suppose we observe two incident cases, or seroconverters, who initially give seronegative donations but subsequently give seropositive donations. The time between donor C's seronegative donation and seropositve donation may have been 20 months, whereas the time between donations for donor D is 7 months. A way to express the incidence rate when subjects are observed for varying amounts of time is to say there were 2 cases per 51 observed person-months (18 + 6 + 20 + 7), or 0.039 cases per person-month. Thus, for each REDS donor, we determined whether or not they were an incident case, and the person-time between their first and last donations.

Table 3 details each marker, the number of donors, the number of observed person-years, the number of incident cases, and the resulting incidence rate, expressed as number of cases per 100,000 person-years. The HCV rate is based on data obtained after the second generation screening test was implemented, so the sample size at this point is much smaller than for other markers. The hepatitis B virus (HBV) incidence rate is based solely on the HBV surface antigen (HBsAg) test. It does not include donors who went from negative to positive on the antibody to hepatitis B core antigen test.

TABLE 3 Preliminary Results of Incidence Analysis[39]

Marker	Number of Donors	Person-Years	Number of Incident Cases	Incidence Rate[a]
Anti-HIV	426,149	421,777	11	2.61
Anti-HTLV-I	426,134	421,767	3	0.71
Anti-HCV	151,708	62,444	4	6.41
HBsAg	426,101	421,734	28	6.64

[a] per 100,000 person-years.

Although the rate for HTLV is based on only 3 incident cases, it is interesting that although the prevalence of HTLV was a little higher than the prevalence of HIV, the incidence of HIV is considerably higher than the incidence of HTLV. The next question is exactly how do you use, or what is the relevance of, an incidence rate? Using HIV as an example, exactly what does 2.61 cases per 100,000 person-years mean?

The incidence rate, when it is a small number such as 2 or 3 per 100,000 person-years, is essentially equivalent to a probability, or risk. So we can say that if the rate is 2.61 per 100,000 person-years, the risk of a person seroconverting within a 1-year period is 1 in 38,000. Normally, we think of

---

[39] See Schreiber et al. (*op cit*) for an updated analysis.

using incidence rates or probabilities to predict the future. That is, we might say that 1 in 38,000 donors will become infected within the next year. But you could also use this figure to say that 1 in 38,000 donors were infected within the past year.

The reason I make this distinction is that in the blood donor setting, the key question really is not "What is the probability that a donor will become infected after donating blood?" The critical question is, "What is the probability that a donor was infected before donating blood?" As I said before, if the donor was infected long enough ago, the serologic test will be positive and the donation will not enter the blood supply. For example, if everyone who was infected more than 6 months ago tests positive, then the question is, "What is the probability that a donor who shows up today to donate blood was infected within the past 6 months?" This is because only this infected donor will test negative and this donation might be used for transfusion.

If we calculated a risk of being infected within the past year to be 1 in 38,000, then the risk of being infected within half of that time, or 6 months, should be half of the risk, or 1 in 76,000. Likewise, we can estimate the risk of being infected within any time frame to be proportional to the risk calculated on a "per year" basis. If we believe that the window period is 45 days, that is, only people who were infected within the past 45 days will have a negative serologic test today, then the risk of one of today's donors being such a person is 1 in 311,000.

On the other hand, remember that we calculated our incidence rate from donors who gave at least 2 donations during our study period. What about first-time donors? It is generally assumed that first-time donors will have higher rates than repeat donors. To see what impact this can have, we can just assume a certain rate for first-time donors relative to that for repeat donors and weight that rate by the percentage of first-time donors in our study.

For example, let us use the observed incidence rate of 2.61 per 100,000 person-years and say the window period is 45 days. If the rate in first-time donors is the same as that in repeat donors, then the risk is 1 in 311,000. But suppose the rate in first-time donors is 50 percent greater than the incidence rate in repeat donors. This means that the rate in first-time donors is about 3.9 per 100,000 person-years. We observed, and other blood donor studies have also reported, that about 21 percent of donations come from first-time donors. So, if we count the 3.9 rate for 21 percent and the 2.6 rate for 79 percent, then the weighted average, when combined with a 45 day window period, adjusts the risk up to 1 in 281,000. Of course, the 50 percent increase was arbitrary. It could be 80 percent, 100 percent or some other value. One previous study estimated that first-time donors would have 1.8 times the incidence rate of repeat donors.[40] Table 4 delineates the impact of varying ratios of incidence rates for first-time versus repeat donors. The point here is that while the risk goes up, it is not overly sensitive to the unknown rate among first-time donors.

TABLE 4 Adjusted Risk of HIV Transmission for First-Time Donors[a]

If the ratio of incidence rates for first-time vs. repeat donors is:	Then the risk of window-period donation is:
1.0	1:311,000
1.5	1:281,000
1.8	1:266,000
2.0	1:257,000

[a] Assumptions are that donors have (1) an incidence rate of 2.61 per 100,000 person-years and (2) a window-period of 45 days, and that (3) 79 percent of donations from repeat donors.

It is interesting to view this risk estimate in light of previous studies. Table 5 presents a partial list of risk estimates in the literature. This is a mixed bag of studies that used different study designs and methodologies to estimate risk. It does show a range of estimates, and depending on what range of variation you are used to working with, you might conclude that they are all in the same ballpark, or you might feel that the estimates are widely disparate. One important factor in looking at risk estimates for HIV is the time frame. As you know, we have had a very dynamic situation with HIV in terms of donor screening and testing.

The studies are listed according to the year that the study ended. The risk estimate from each study is multiplied by 18,000,000, which is the number of donations or units that are collected each year in the United States, to get the number of window-period donations that would be expected to enter the blood supply each year. There appears to be a trend of decreasing risk with time; that is, more recent risk estimates appear to be lower than older risk estimates. This downward trend over time is what you would expect if you were decreasing the incidence rate (by effective donor screening) and/or decreasing the window period (by improved HIV tests).

---

[40] Cumming, PD, EL Wallace, JB Schorr, RY Dodd (1989). Exposure of patients to human immunodeficiency virus through the transfusion of blood components that test antibody-negative. *New England Journal of Medicine, 321(14):* 941–946. Comment in *New England Journal of Medicine, 322(12):* 850–851.

TABLE 5 Risk of a Window-Period Donation Due to a Seroconverting HIV-Positive Donor: Estimates from Previous Studies

Source	Study Dates	Risk Estimate	No. of Window-Period Donations Expected
Ward et al.[41]	1986–1987	1:38,000	474
Kleinman and Second[42]	1986–1987	1:68,000	265
Cumming et al.[43]	1985–1987	1:153,000	118
Cohen et al.[44]	1985–1989	1:36,000	500
Busch et al.[45]	1987–1989	1:61,000	295
Kleinman[46]	1988–1989	1:106,000	170
Nelson et al.[47]	1985–1991	1:60,000	300
Petersen et al.[48]	1988–1991	1:220,000	82
REDS[49]	1991–1992	1:257,000	70
Vyas et al.[50]	1987–1993	1:160,000	112

Finally, Table 6 points out how the incidence rate can be used to help assess the impact of shortening a window period, again using HIV as an example. It might be that there is uncertainty or controversy over the total length of the window period. Is it 45 days, or 60 days, or 30 days? However,

---

[41]Ward, JW, SD Holmberg, JR Allen, DL Cohn, et al. (1988). Transmission of human immunodeficiency virus (HIV) by blood transfusions screened as negative for HIV antibody. *New England Journal of Medicine, 318(8):* 473–478.

[42]Kleinman, S and K Second (1988). Risk of human immunodeficiency virus (HIV) transmission by anti-HIV negative blood: Estimates using the lookback methodology. *Transfusion, 28:* 499–501.

[43]Cumming et al. (1989), *op cit.*

[44]Cohen, ND, A Munoz, BA Reitz, PK Ness et al. (1989). transmission of retroviruses by transfusion of screened blood in patients undergoing cardiac surgery. *New England Journal of Medicine, 320(18):* 1172–1176.

[45]Busch, MP, BE Eble, H Khayam-Bashi, D Heilbron et al. (1991). Evaluation of screened blood donations for human immunodeficiency virus type 1 infection by culture and DNA amplification of pooled cells. *New England Journal of Medicine, 325(1):* 1–5.

[46]Unpublished.

[47]Nelson, KE, JG Donahue, A Munoz, ND Cohen et al. (1992). transmission of retroviruses from seronegative donors by transfusion during cardiac surgery. A multicenter study of HIV-1 and HTLV-I/II infections. *Annals of Internal Medicine, 117(7):* 554–559.

[48]Petersen, L, MP Busch, G Satten, R Dodd et al. (1993). Narrowing the window period with a third generation anti-HIV-1-2 enzyme immunoassay: relevance to P24 antigen screening of blood donors in the United States [abstract]. *International Conference on AIDS, 9(2):* 717.

[49]See Schreiber et al. (*op cit*) for an updated analysis.

[50]Vyas, GN, BD Rawal, G Babu, MP Busch (1994). Diminishing risk of HIV infection from transfusion of seronegative blood [abstract]. *Transfusion, 34(Suppl.):* 63S.

regardless of the total window-period length, it might be possible to estimate how many days sooner a new test will detect HIV antibodies. For example, we might not know whether the window period is 30 or 60 days, but we might determine that a new test shortens the window period, whatever it is, by say 5 days. If we use the REDS incidence rate and make the other usual assumptions, we can estimate that shortening the window period by 5 days will detect between 8 and 13 HIV-infected donations that otherwise would have tested negative. The same approach could be applied to any other shortening of the window period. This information helps estimate the yield or benefit of a new test, which then might be incorporated into a cost-benefit analysis of a proposed new test.

TABLE 6 Impact of Shortening the HIV Window Period[a]

If the window period is shortened by:	Then the number of additional HIV-infected donations detected will be:
1 day	2–3
2 days	3–5
3 days	5–8
4 days	6–10
5 days	8–13
10 days	16–26

[a] Assumptions are (1) a donor incidence rate of 2.61 per 100,000 person-years, (2) 79 percent of donations are from repeat donors, (3) first-time donors have 2.0 times the incidence rate, and (4) there are 18 million donations[51]

In conclusion, while the prevalence of seropositive donations is relevant, especially in a broad public health context, it is really at best an indirect measure of risk to the blood supply. The incidence rate, which we were able to calculate because we have information that links together a donor's multiple donations over time, is a better measure of risk (specifically transfusion-associated risk) because it estimates the risk of recent infection.

We saw how the risk of donation during an infectious window period depends directly, proportionately, and equally on the incidence rate and the length of the window period and how the incidence rate can be used to assess the impact, or yield, or benefit of shortening the window period. I have used

---

[51] See Schreiber et al. (*op cit*) for an updated analysis.

HIV as an example, but the same points and same methods can be applied to other infectious diseases as well. We are currently in the process of estimating demographic-specific incidence rates. I think it will be interesting to see if the same demographic patterns that have been observed in the prevalence of infectious disease markers hold for the incidence rates.

Finally, REDS will continue to monitor and report on changes with time, and will incorporate results from the other REDS components, such as the special donor surveys, as part of its mission to monitor the safety of the U.S. blood supply.

CDC Surveillance of Donors

Eve M. Lackritz

Surveillance is the ongoing and systematic collection, analysis, and interpretation of health data. The Centers for Disease Control and Prevention (CDC) monitors the transmission of transfusion-transmitted diseases through these ongoing data collection systems. Different branches and divisions at CDC, including the Division of HIV/AIDS Prevention, have their own surveillance activities. Surveillance provides information for action: decision making, policy development, and development of prevention strategies.

Within the Division of HIV/AIDS Prevention, several branches have surveillance activities to monitor the transmission of HIV by blood transfusion. The Surveillance Branch manages the HIV/AIDS Reporting System, which receives reports of all patients with AIDS, including those who were infected from screened blood or blood products. In addition to managing the surveillance system, the Surveillance Branch conducts special studies to follow-up on AIDS cases that were reported to have been transmitted by transfusion of screened blood.

The HIV Seroepidemiology Branch is responsible for two surveillance projects that I would like to discuss. One study collects information on all blood donations from 19 of the 45 American Red Cross blood services regions. The second study, the CDC HIV Blood Donor Study, involves interviewing HIV-positive blood donors from 20 different U.S. blood centers across the country and maintaining a repository of serum and cell samples from these donors. The blood centers in the interview study are not the same as those in the Red Cross study.

The collaborative study with the American Red Cross collects information on approximately 2 million donations each year from 19 Red Cross regions. These regions were selected because they have compatible computerized data management systems, thus allowing data from different regions to be merged and analyzed. Information collected on each donation includes donor demographic information, whether the donor was a first-time or repeat donor, the dates of the most recent and previous donations, and whether the donor elected to confidentially exclude his or her donation from being transfused (the confidential unit exclusion system, or CUE). All laboratory test results of these donations are also included in the database. The regional blood centers voluntarily forward their data to the American Red Cross, which then cleans the dataset and forwards it to CDC.

This dataset gives us a great deal of information that we use in policy-making and decision-making. For example, the requirement to test all blood donations for syphilis has been maintained because the syphilis test is a surrogate marker for HIV risk behaviors. A surrogate test removes donations by HIV-infected volunteers donating during the window period of seronegativity that would otherwise not be detected by routine HIV testing. Analysis of the Red Cross data allowed us to evaluate the cost and effectiveness of syphilis testing as a surrogate marker for HIV window period donations. We have also used the Red Cross dataset to evaluate the effectiveness of the confidential unit exclusion system and more recently the risk of HIV transmission by screened blood in the United States.

The second surveillance project conducted by the HIV Seroepidemiology Branch is the CDC HIV Blood Donor Study. Twenty U.S. blood centers participate in this project. These centers tend to have more HIV-positive donors than other areas. Participating blood centers contact all blood donors who test positive for HIV and request that they return to the center to be informed of their HIV test results and counseled. At the counseling visit, the centers ask the donor to participate in a standardized interview as part of the CDC study.

The donor interview takes about an hour to complete. Donors are asked about their HIV risk behaviors and their motivations for donation. CDC also receives laboratory test results of these donations. Partner testing is offered, as is a follow-up interview for those who don't have any identified risks for HIV. Donors often do not discover that their partners are HIV positive or identify other risk factors until after the donor notification and counseling session. A blood sample is collected at the time of the interview for the serum and cell repository, which has become a very valuable research tool.

We have used information obtained from the CDC HIV Blood Donor Study for several different purposes. First, we have evaluated trends in risk behaviors among HIV-positive donors and have identified methods to improve predonation interviews and the donor deferral system. We have investigated such as issues as whether donors were given enough privacy during predonation interviews and why donors with known risk behaviors donated blood. Second, we have studied the effect of donor incentives by evaluating the motivations and risk characteristics of HIV-positive blood donors. Third, the study has served as a means of monitoring for HIV-2 in the blood supply. Fourth, we have used the serum and cell repository to monitor for the introduction of rare HIV subtypes into the blood supply and to ensure that current HIV tests are detecting rare HIV variants.

Currently, we are examining whether HIV-seropositive individuals are donating blood in order to be tested for HIV. The study of test-seeking behavior is particularly important because of the recent licensure of the p24 antigen test. We estimate that, among the approximately 12 million donations made in the United States each year, 7 to 10 donations will be HIV antigen positive and antibody negative. If individuals at risk for HIV infection donate blood to receive this special HIV test, the benefits of antigen testing may be offset by an increase in donations from donors at high risk for HIV infection. Therefore, monitoring this "magnet effect" is critical.

These ongoing surveillance projects allow us to monitor trends in transmission of HIV by transfusion and risk behaviors among blood donors. However, CDC also stays poised to deal with new and uncharacterized threats to the blood supply through special investigations and outbreak investigations. These allow CDC to respond rapidly to new or emerging diseases or adverse events. A recent example of one of these special investigations is the investigation of HIV Group O, an HIV variant potentially not detected by routine HIV antibody screening. CDC collaborated with the Retrovirus Epidemiology Donor Study (REDS) and other study groups to retest blood donations that had positive and indeterminate HIV Western blot results and negative EIA results with high optical density readings. Other special studies include collaborative look-back investigations to determine the length of the HIV infectious window period and the risk of HIV transmission by screened blood. Currently, we are developing an evaluation of the benefit, cost, and magnet effect of HIV p24 antigen testing.

CDC is not a regulatory agency; we work through collaboration and consensus building to collect and analyze information to promote public health in the United States.

DISCUSSION

James Allen: Let me initiate the discussion by asking about costs versus benefits. We are in a cost-crunching time right now. Can we justify the continued relatively high cost of these programs in terms of what we are getting from them?

Thomas Zuck: The current funding level of REDS should not be sustained beyond the defined period of 1998. We are in the process now of calculating how much it will cost to keep the system in place without the continuing acquisition of new data and without additional physical examinations of the HTLV-infected cohort. The cost has been about $4 million a year over the 9 years of the study. For about 1/10 of that we can keep the surveillance part intact. If you consider the costs of AIDS and hepatitis C infection, then that is a fairly low price to pay in relation to better than $1 billion of health care.

James Allen: Five years from now we will be well beyond the current data. We will have the laboratory repository but one would then have to question the utility of data that are 5 or more years old.

Thomas Zuck: Another aspect of the database that may be equally as important is its ability to validate new technologies. There will be a day, probably within the next decade, when polymerase chain reaction (PCR) will be automated and the specificity problem will have been sorted out. Maybe it will be ligase chain reactions instead of PCR, but a genetic technology will be available within a decade. Those repositories are enormously valuable to validate the quality, specificity, and sensitivity of those tests.

Eve Lackritz: There is also a difference between actual risk and perceived risk. What often drives blood safety policy and programs is the public perception that the blood supply is not safe. In terms of HIV, the blood supply is very safe, but the public remains concerned. We need to continue to monitor the safety of the blood supply, but we must also identify ways to more effectively communicate our findings to the public.

Paul McCurdy: Many people in the audience know that in the late 1970's the National Heart, Lung and Blood Institute sponsored a transfusion transmitted virus study, the so-called TTV study. As part of that study a repository was established that has been used to look at prevention of hepatitis C virus transmission by antibody testing. It is now being used to look at hepatitis G virus which has relatively recently been described and probably will be used to examine some of the antigen testing procedures. The REDS repository and data may turn out to be equally valuable for unknown reasons sometime in the future.

Thomas Zuck: One of the major advantages of the TTV study is that the TTV data are linked to recipients, and that makes it uniquely valuable. One of the weaknesses of REDS is that we don't have recipient linkages. Now, we could go back and create them, because the data are all encrypted, but the great strength of TTV is that it has that recipient linkage.

Paul McCurdy: The transfusion safety study also had a repository and a lot of data.

Thomas Zuck: Again, however, they were unlinked to recipients. The uniqueness of TTV is the recipient linkage.

Lew Barker: These sorts of studies are extraordinarily valuable, but I wonder how to maintain surveillance as cost-effectively as possible because it is going to continue to be important, and how to maintain the ability to look at new technologies relatively quickly and efficiently.

Thomas Zuck: That is the great value of the repositories. If a strategy appears (and we don't know what kind of genomic analysis is going to come down the line), then the REDS repositories will be the fastest place to go to find the answer to new technologies or emerging viruses.

Eve Lackritz: I think the repositories are going to become increasingly important, and we are putting more of our emphasis on that. There are ways to streamline the budget, but notifying donors and bringing them in for interviews and sample collection are labor-intensive activities.

Harold Sox: I was part of the Institute of Medicine Committee that produced *HIV and the Blood Supply*, and back in 1983 there was information, like a ligand, but there was no receptor over at the Food and Drug Administration (FDA). You mentioned that you are a surveillance agency, not a regulatory agency. Could you tell us whether that receptor is in place now and whether the internal workings of the cell, just to extend the analogy, are such that the signal gets transduced to take some action?

Eve Lackritz: We collect information for the purpose of taking action. We communicate regularly with FDA through a Public Health Service (PHS) conference call that FDA coordinates twice a month. When we realize available information is limited, other people are contacted to provide additional information to that forum. Thus, there is a system in place. For example, we routinely do analyses for Blood Products Advisory Committee meetings. Whenever an issue comes up, we are poised to respond with the appropriate dataset, and vice versa. If we receive a report of an emerging disease or adverse event, we contact FDA. The ties are very strong, and it has been a good relationship.

William Sherwood: Repositories have limitations. We had a repository of samples from hemophiliacs. It wasn't all in one place, but the libraries of sera went back to the 1950s. Yet they couldn't be used. We learned in 1985 that at least 20 percent of hemophiliacs were infected with HIV before we even knew that there was a such a virus, and far more were infected before we had a test. You cannot really use these repositories until you have a test.

Eve Lackritz: The other important thing is that we have interviews from these donors. AIDS reporting started before an etiologic agent had been identified. You can start doing epidemiology without a known test, and our existing systems are flexible enough that we can modify them and capture those events, using a new case definition if need be. Also, having repositories in place allows for a more rapid response to a new problem, such as when we used peptide assays to study Group O in the U.S. blood supply.

Thomas Zuck: You really cannot get prevalence data without a test, and lack of a test was what was confounding things in the early 1980s. No one thought that the prevalence was as high as it was when we started asking the high-risk questions. You really need a test to get a handle on prevalence. That was the key element missing in 1983 and 1984.

Surveillance of Recipients

James R. Allen

Our session today is titled Guarding the Blood Supply. Since all the presentations focus on the role of data collection through surveillance to detect potential problems rather than data developed through special studies or research, I am going to begin my remarks with a short exegesis on surveillance.

Surveillance is quite different from special studies or research. Special studies start with a specific hypothesis that is to be tested. The studies are focused, are conducted in a fairly defined population, and most often within a closed time frame. Special studies rely on defined data elements gathered to form a fairly rigid data set, and the methodology is well established to insure that the data collected are accurate and reliable, and that they can be confirmed.

Surveillance on the other hand is much more nebulous. The intent is to identify a problem, not to fully study it. Surveillance, therefore, has characteristics very different from those of special studies or research. Surveillance is a data-gathering system, whether active or passive. Most surveillance systems are passive; that is, they rely on observations and reports of people who may not recognize that they are part of a routine data collection system. The individual reports are collected in a central repository, whether it be at the local or state health department, the Centers for Disease Control and Prevention (CDC), a blood collection center, or any other organization that may be collecting the information.

Surveillance systems may use defined methods or they may simply rely on random reports being generated and sent in. The population under surveillance is often open and may change over time for various reasons. The population is often not well-defined, even when there is a specific target population. Bruce Evatt will address surveillance in special populations, people with hemophilia in particular. This is a small well-defined population, but I think Bruce will readily acknowledge that there are many people with hemophilia who may be outside of the defined population system, and that there may be events going on with them that do not get reported back in routinely.

The data gathered through a surveillance system most often are highly restricted, since it is not practical to collect a large amount of information, especially through a passive surveillance system. The primary data collected are demographic, the specific event of interest, and a limited set of data about the circumstances that surround the event or important laboratory findings. Also, surveillance systems are often open-ended, since there is no defined time frame within which the study is going to be completed. Surveillance is a continuing process that forms a rolling database.

Although that brief discussion provides the essence of surveillance systems, I want to mention two other characteristics that are extremely important to successful surveillance. First, somebody has to be responsible for analyzing or looking at the data on a regular basis. Too often a surveillance system may have data entered into a database system on a continuing basis but never have that wealth of information analyzed or looked at critically by a human being who is asking questions, plotting trends, and trying to make sense out of the data. The data may get dumped into tables. They may be published or made available in various formats, but nobody really looks at the data, thinks about them, asks questions, and tries to make sense out of them. Second, the final component of surveillance is for that data or information to be disseminated to those who need to know and who can act on the data. If the data are reported to a surveillance system but remain in a repository and are not disseminated to those who can act on it, they do not do any good.

I will now turn to the focus of today's meeting—recipients of blood and blood products. We will define recipients for this purpose as being a person who has received an infusion of any blood or blood component as part of his or her therapy. We are not talking about the special populations or people with a defined disease or a defined situation. We are talking about the general population here.

The notion that if you don't know where you are going, any road will get you there epitomizes the problem that we have with defining surveillance for disease or for adverse events in a population. There are subcomponents that we can break out. The time course of the event or presumed event is extremely important. For example, doing surveillance for transfusion reaction is relatively easy. There is a short time course from the time of infusion to the time at which the event occurs, the patient is usually still on site, and it is a clinical event that is fairly well recognized.

We then have the intermediate time course problems, such as transfusion-associated hepatitis, and there may be either active or passive surveillance systems for monitoring what is happening. We are talking about a time event of 6 to 8 months. There may be a clinical event or it may be subclinical, but we have good laboratory markers for many of the hepatitis types that are transfusion transmitted. The clinicians involved may report back to the blood banking system, or the blood banking system may have an active system in place, or we may set up special studies if we have particular concerns and want to look at the situation very intensively with a very sophisticated study for a relatively short period of time.

What about surveillance for longer-term events, however, or events that are ill defined? This becomes more difficult. The paradigm that we can use is what we now know to be transfusion-transmitted human immunodeficiency virus (HIV) infection occurring in the early 1980s. The first cases of AIDS were recognized in mid-1981, and were reported to CDC. The first thing that had to be done was to put together the clinical parameters and then the immunologic parameters. Over the first 3 to 6 months, CDC, health departments, and clinicians around the country did a superb job of assembling the basic epidemiologic parameters. By mid-1982, just 12 months after the recognition of the epidemic, we understood the potential for AIDS to be transfusion transmitted.

At CDC we recognized that we had this unusual clinical condition in people with hemophilia. But how did we know it was the same disease in all of them inasmuch as people with hemophilia have a lot of other events occurring to them? They are not your standard patient population, and the disease was ill defined. We had no lab markers. Yet, the system began to respond immediately. We became aware of the potential for transfusion-transmitted diseases, and when the first reports did reach CDC that fall, the investigations began to try to get all the pieces of information that were going to be used to confirm that event.

It was late November 1982, when the first report came into CDC of an infant who became ill, when the information began to fall into place. At that time, even though we had a number of children from New York and New Jersey in particular who had a condition that seemed to be a pediatric AIDS-like condition, no one had yet formally accepted that children got AIDS. There had not been a case report of pediatric AIDS published in the *Morbidity and Mortality Weekly Report* or anywhere else at that point. We had all these unusual events that were coming together, and we had to try to sort them out and put them together. It was remarkable that the information was obtained as efficiently and rapidly as it was, and that the pieces of the puzzle were able to be put together extremely well, such that by early 1983 we had a fairly clear picture of the outline for the puzzle, even though we didn't have all of the center of the puzzle filled in.

In retrospect, could we have done better on that? I don't think we could have done much better in terms of rapidly recognizing an unexpected or unpredictable event with a pathogen that was brand new and with a disease that was ill defined in the absence of any specific laboratory markers.

Could we have done better in terms of getting close cooperation and collaboration among all the participants, the CDC, the National Institutes of Health, the Food and Drug Administration, the blood collection centers, hospitals, and various other aspects of the health care system? Yes, in retrospect, that might have worked more smoothly. Nonetheless, given the diversity of our system, our concern about the rights of individual people and confidentiality of patient records, and the absence of any preexisting collaborative system, it still worked relatively smoothly, and we were able to get a lot of answers very quickly.

What then might we learn in terms of lessons for today? Can we put a more formalized surveillance system into place for transfusion recipients, one that will get information back to us rapidly, help us to identify either known or unknown problems in the future? If you really want to do that, you have to have an active tracking system for following up transfusion recipients, to gather clinical information and blood samples for additional testing and placement in a repository. However, it is not feasible, nor is it necessary. It would be extremely expensive, and it would not be cost-effective.

For the known problems, it is important that we continue to publish information about current events and trends and to be certain that clinicians as well as health officials, blood banking officials, and federal government officials are all aware of that information. We need to be very aggressive at instituting special studies as appropriate.

We need a strong general database at all levels, particularly computer-based patient records. One of the issues related to transfusion-associated investigations in the early 1980s was trying to get back to the patient record to determine if that patient did in fact receive that unit of blood. The unit would have been signed out by the blood bank, but there would be no record in the medical record that the unit was ever returned back to the blood bank. We often couldn't confirm that the patient received that unit of blood.

We need much stronger linkages between the blood collection center, the hospital transfusion service, and the patient record. We need to refine the linkage as one gets beyond the transfusion service to the patient record, the clinician, or the current physician of record if we are really going to do a good job of general surveillance. Over the next 5 to 10 years, as we move to managed care, some of these issues will begin to be addressed.

We will need to have long-term maintenance of the record. How long is long enough? If you go back a decade, medical records will be boxed up and not available if the patient hasn't come into the system in the preceding 5 or 6 years. Records should be maintained for at least 10 years, and maybe 15 years, for us to be able to go back and access patient and transfusion records.

Surveillance for unknown problems begins with having a high curiosity level and a high index of suspicion and being willing to get back to an appropriate reporting or communication source very early on. It obviously means that it must be incumbent on the public health system that is receiving that report to make an appropriate analysis and pass it up through the system. I am very concerned about what is happening to our state and local public health agencies, as well as at the federal level, given the budget and personnel cuts that are coming.

Finally, it is possible to get useful information out of large surveillance systems that are in place for other reasons. For example, CDC has a hospital-based record system, the National Nosocomial Infection Study, intended to look at infections occurring in hospitals. This is a multiple-hospital reporting system that has been used in the past to detect and evaluate problems with contamination of large-volume parenteral fluids. In about 1970, a nationwide outbreak occurred via the fluids distributed by one manufacturer, and even with the small neophyte system at CDC then, we got a glimmer of the problem. The CDC system picked up the unusual pattern of infections reported, and made queries to other hospitals that then confirmed the pattern. When CDC later did much more intensive analyses using its surveillance system, the data were there. The problem could have been detected had CDC been looking at the data promptly and in exactly the right manner. It is intriguing what can be done with these systems if you have the resources to look at the information that is there and that is being reported.

Might such a system be helpful in transfusion-transmitted diseases? It all depends. If you are getting sick from infusion of large-volume parenteral fluids, that is occurring very proximate to the hospitalization. However, with transfusion-transmitted infections we are looking at events that occur months to years afterward. There isn't any way of easily getting those records back into the hospital-based system. Nonetheless, I think models that might be appropriate in the future are available, but they will be costly. In summary, we are much better off going with a general awareness and a much less structured system, similar to what we had in the early 1980s. That system worked very well.

DISCUSSION

Harold Sox: You mentioned that an ongoing surveillance system was too expensive. Has there been a thorough cost-effectiveness analysis of a wide variety of different approaches to implementing a screening process?

James Allen: When I said that it would be too expensive, I was talking about an active system that is specifically trying to get back information. That would be extremely difficult and very costly, with very little useful information coming back. I am not aware of any cost analyses of that.

Scott Wetterhall: If you have a database or a serum repository but you don't have a disease, there is nothing to survey at that point. There may be benefits in terms of maintaining serum repositories in terms of obtaining additional information once a disease has been recognized. Clearly, what is relevant for this group, given that the safety of the blood supply is the issue, is that you need a diagnostic test. You are maintaining a system, and yet you don't have anything that you are measuring. It is really only in a retrospective sense that it may provide you with information.

Harold Sox: Suppose you are worried about a disease occurring that would have the same catastrophic effects that AIDS did. You could do a model which would basically assume the disease you were looking for. The only reason for doing the surveillance would be to detect something as bad as AIDS and then trying to get a handle on what different levels of surveillance might cost and what the benefits would be. Without that type of analysis we run the risk that we will repeat the AIDS history.

William Sherwood: We know from the repositories that were tested in 1985 that the AIDS virus entered the hemophiliac population in about 1978. If we had all the money in the world, what surveillance program could we have put in place in 1978 to prevent what happened?

Bruce Evatt: The key is that the surveillance program should be coupled to other programs. But surveillance programs of high-risk groups are extremely expensive. If surveillance is part of an ongoing program that deals with other issues and is integrated into those programs, then it is very feasible to do. But with a surveillance system, it is somebody's responsibility to examine for unknown events.

Repositories do no good unless you have a test, but here we are not talking about repositories. We are talking about clinical events that occur out of the usual occurrence. Therefore, ongoing programs that deal with that issue would have picked this up. I can tell you with HIV in the early 1980s the surveillance program that helped us was the pentamidine investicational new drug (IND) application. That is where we found all the early cases of HIV infection among both hemophiliacs and transfusion recipients. Because the requests all came to us, we used that file to identify new patients for whom there were no known no risk factors. That is how we identified the those cases. If we hadn't had the IND for pentamidine and if pentamidine wasn't used to treat *Pneumocystis carinii* pneumonia, we wouldn't have identified

AIDS in hemophiliacs, because most of the times when we investigated AIDS among hemophilia patients or transfusion recipients, their physicians had no idea that these people had AIDS. We ended up informing the hemophilia treatment center doctors that these patients probably had AIDS, and that it was a new disease.

What was useful for us was the presence of a system, a data collection system that existed for another purpose. You must identify such information collection systems that might be useful and that can be justified on an ongoing basis for some other purpose, plug into those systems, and make it somebody's responsibility to look for unusual clinical events. This is because the first occurrences of new diseases will not be discovered by a test that you can use to go to a repository. It is going to be unusual clinical events that point the direction to a new syndrome that is out of the ordinary, and that means you have to know the background levels of such events. You must know the incidence of those unusual events, and you must look for changes in trends. That is the form that surveillance of these kinds of problems is going to have to take. Setting up a surveillance program for the purpose of surveillance at $4 million a year is a big waste of money. It must be incorporated into the standard ongoing programs for which data are being collected for other reasons. You must have somebody looking at one or two questions that identify the unusual risk.

James Allen: What you just described there is a key point that we have made over and over, and that is that somebody must be looking at the data, interpreting them, and getting them out where they will be useful. Data systems by themselves aren't very useful if nobody is looking at them.

CDC Surveillance of High-Risk Recipients

Bruce Evatt

Serum repositories have been collected in the past, but few have been very helpful in retrospect. Ongoing information collection is the most useful source of information in the identification of emerging situations involving blood-borne infections.

Congress has given the Centers for Disease Control and Prevention (CDC) the responsibility to develop a long-term program for the prevention of the complications of hemophilia. This program consists of several phases. First, we are to define the scope of the complications within the hemophilia population. The second task is to assess prevention opportunities for the major complications. Finally, CDC is to design prevention programs, develop resources to address those complications, and evaluate whether these programs are clinically effective and cost-effective.

Hemophilia is an extremely expensive disease. It costs about $1 billion a year to care for approximately 17,000 patients. Thus, if a 10 percent improvement in the effectiveness and efficiency of the programs can be made, an improvement in the health care delivery system for the individual hemophilia patient will occur at a considerable savings of health care resources.

In the early 1980s we thought that most of this population was cared for primarily by hemophilia treatment centers. We discovered that this wasn't the case when we began to examine mortality data collected from surveys of the hemophilia treatment centers. We found that when these data were compared with the death certificate data, only about two-thirds of the hemophilia patients were within hemophilia treatment centers. Another one-third were outside those centers. Nothing was known of the source of their care or the nature of their disease. Thus, the first part of the system was to define the hemophilia population, where they received their care, and the nature of their complications before we could prioritize the complications.

The present hemophilia surveillance system was designed to identify this population. This surveillance system is unique in that there are no existing surveillance models for chronic diseases of low incidence. There are surveillance models for acute infectious diseases and chronic diseases of high incidence such as diabetes.

This is not an inexpensive system, nor is it a system that has universal application. Likewise, it is not a system that needs to last indefinitely. This system was directed at six states, which contain about 25 percent of the supposed hemophilia population. They are Massachusetts, New York, Georgia, Louisiana, Colorado, and Oklahoma.

This system was designed to characterize the distribution of the types of hemophilia, the severity, the resource utilization, the complications, and the level of joint disease as well as other aspects of hemophilia. Confidentiality is rigidly enforced. It was much more than the standard annual infectious disease surveillance system. It consists of an annual retrospective chart review of all the hemophilia patients within the six states. Most of the patients would be identified in hemophilia treatment centers. A very important part of the study, however, was to define individuals who did not receive their care from hemophilia treatment centers. It is easy to obtain information from organized hemophilia treatment centers, but very difficult to track down and identify a patient outside hemophilia treatment centers. Nonetheless, the goal of this system is to identify 100 percent of the patients in these states. All six state health departments have requested that hemophilia be a reportable disease in order to facilitate case finding.

In addition, patients are also identified with the aid of the local hemophilia chapters, people who supply clotting factor information; pharmacies, hematologists, clinical record systems, hospitals and physicians' offices also supply patient information. Laboratories report any patients with Factor VIII or IX below the level of 30 percent. All are investigated, so that all patients will be identified.

The data collection consists of demographics, source of care, hospital issues such as the hemophilia type and severity, the number of bleeds, the factor used, inhibitors, and the number on prophylaxis. More importantly, surveillance information on viral infections, joint disease, HIV status, and any new infections will be gathered to track emerging trends. We will also document all hospitalizations, including the dates and diagnoses, as well as other kinds of infections, such as sepsis, and other complications of transfusions as part of this database. Currently we have 2 years of data in the database. These data are used by the local community as well as being transported electronically to a centralized database at CDC.

We are particularly interested in identifying viral infections with this system. We should have the ability to identify both acute and chronic hepatitis B virus (HBV) infections, acute and chronic hepatitis C virus (HCV) infections, acute hepatitis A virus (HAV) infections, and HIV seroconversions. Because this is designed to be a retrospective review of information on these patients, it will not detect infections quickly in any individual patient. We will be able to detect unusual syndromes in individual hemophilia patients, as well as trends in infections. If a number of unusual diagnoses occur clinically we will be able to detect these.

Approximately 115 hemophilia treatment centers in the United States currently care for about 14,000 individuals with hemophilia A and B and another 3,000 or 4,000 individuals with von Willebrand's disease. We currently finance these hemophilia treatment centers for prevention activities. The Health Resources and Services Administration provides these centers with another $5 million a year for health care services.

We want to broaden the scope of prevention activities in these centers to include studies of prevention interventions for the complications of hemophilia, including blood-borne infections. As part of that we will require a data collection system to help us determine whether our prevention programs make a difference in health outcome.

The two highest priorities for us are reducing the level of joint disease in the community and monitoring blood safety. The data collection system needs to be simple and ongoing. We are designing a universal data collection system that will become part of the clinical activities of all of those 115 hemophilia treatment centers. Such a system would monitor two-thirds of the U.S. hemophilia population. This data collection system would be prospective, would assess the level of hemophilia care that is being provided, and would identify issues for specific studies.

Time constraints limit the amount of data collection, and we recognize that. We need to address the amount of data that are available and the type of collection instrument that we will use. We must consider routine practice within the hemophilia treatment center and create a data collection system that is useful to those centers as a whole.

The initial targets will be hepatitis viruses and HIV. Those are of major concern to the hemophilia community and must be addressed. The data to be collected will include the basic clinical profile, annual viral testing for the known viruses, and other issues of interest. In the first year we will only be able to measure prevalence rates. In subsequent years we will be able to follow incidence rates in this population. The occurrence of acute cases of HCV infection, HBV infection, and HIV infection will trigger specific investigations to ascertain if these infections were acquired through blood and blood products. We will do this in collaboration with the Food and Drug Administration and the National Institutes of Health.

This surveillance program is to be implemented within the coming year. Realistically it will take a year to get the program in place. If FDA and the National Heart, Lung and Blood Institute (NHLBI) feel that more frequent reporting is necessary, we can incorporate that into the system design. In summary this system will identify new infections to be investigated for the source of infection. Also, the system will be used to monitor the regional trends and variations in blood-borne infections.

Finally, I would like to talk very briefly about the potential risk of Creutzfeldt-Jakob disease (CJD) being transmitted in blood products. Currently there is no evidence that it is transmitted in blood products. However, the risk cannot be assessed with any degree of accuracy. It is felt by everyone to be extremely low, if at all, and remains a theoretical risk at best. The troublesome thing is that it can be transferred to experimental animals by a transmittable agent, and the agent is present within the blood of the patients with CJD. That makes it a theoretical risk. The epidemiologic question is how do you do surveillance on a disease that has an incubation period of 20 to 30 years? It is not impossible, but it doesn't lead to any kind of ideal solution where you ascertain the risk very quickly. The hemophilia community is quite concerned about CJD, and they are anxious to have answers as soon as possible. The only way we can reasonably approach this problem is with a special study.

Currently, 400 deaths occur annually in the hemophilia community in the United States. About 300 of these are caused by AIDS; the other 100 are caused by non-AIDS-related events. Of the 300 who die from AIDS, about 30 to 50 have central nervous system (CNS) AIDS. The hemophilia population has been routinely receiving concentrates for 20 and 25 years now. We would thus expect that if CJD was caused by a transmittable agent in blood products, you might be seeing cases now in individuals with hemophilia. The only condition that could be misdiagnosed would be individuals who have been diagnosed as having CNS AIDS. I have received several letters from individual physicians who treated hemophilia patients who had died with CNS AIDS before the publicity on CJD. There were no autopsies and no post-mortem examinations of these patients. Now these physicians are wondering if these might have been possible cases of CJD.

It is this kind of rumor that spreads quite quickly in the hemophilia population because it is a very small, closed community. Both the physicians and the hemophilia patients now agree that the only solution to this is to try to obtain as many postmortem examinations as possible in individuals who die with CNS AIDS over the next several years. We have established a collaborative project between ourselves and Dr. De Arman at the University of California, San Francisco, the various hemophilia treatment centers, FDA, and NIH, as well as the various peer groups from the hemophilia population. We hope to obtain 10 to 15 brains per year for this study.

The basic design of this study is to obtain permission at the time of death to remove the brain for a CNS autopsy. One-centimeter cubed biopsy specimens will be removed from the frontal, midparietal, and cerebellar regions and frozen. The remainder of brain will be placed in formalin for 2 weeks.

These specimens will then will receive a routine pathologic workup for dementia and an examination for the prion protein. Suspect cases will be reviewed by a panel of neuropathologists selected by ourselves, NIH, and FDA. A single case of CJD under the age of 40 would be very significant. A CJD case in an individual over the age of 40 could mean that we must continue this study, since a case of CJD in an older person won't carry the same weight as one in someone who is young.

In summary, the collection systems, with the exception of CJD, which is a special study, are part of a national program designed to assist in lowering the complications of hemophilia. These data collection tools, however, can also be utilized very effectively to monitor blood-borne infections in this community and for observing whether there is any new incidence of unusual diseases. It may be that the only way that we will be able to obtain the information needed to monitor blood safety for relatively rare events or unknown events in a cost-effective manner.

DISCUSSION

Paul Russell: What evidence do you have that it takes 20 or 30 years for Creutzfeldt-Jakob disease to be manifested?

Bruce Evatt: It comes from several types of data. Some of it is from studies of cannibals in terms of kuru and other types of slow virus diseases. Certainly, the delay in onset was much shorter than 20 to 30 years in the cases of growth hormone-induced transmission. Thus, the delay is probably related to the dose of the agent, although it is probably related to other issues as well.

David Rothman: When you made hemophilia a reportable disease, did you already know all about stigma? Do you have any built-in patient confidentially in any of these surveillance efforts?

Bruce Evatt: Yes, we worried about a reaction from the hemophilia community. You have to understand that one of the issues that you deal with, confidentiality, is of utmost importance in this community, especially as it concerns HIV and AIDS. One of the problems we had during the 1980s was the fact that the hemophilia population didn't want to be identified. There was no registry of hemophilia patients. Even if you wanted to, you could not have notified them of risks associated with a new disease because they didn't want their names obtained by anybody. The lack of a registry in the hemophilia community has been a major issue. Obtaining a complete accounting of all individuals with hemophilia in the six states has been accomplished very successfully. We managed this in two ways.

First, the state health departments are the only entities that have the names. They have the right to do that in all of these states. They all have normal procedures to keep names confidential. In many states people in state health departments can go to jail for breaking confidentiality. Thus, they have a track record of maintaining confidentiality over a long period of time; that reassures people. Furthermore, there was an encryption of the identifiers. We do not know who, where, or what they are. It is to maintain a unique identifier for the database so that they can be followed subsequently by the state health department.

The second way this was managed was that personnel from the state health departments met with the hemophilia chapters to explain the study. They told the chapters how the study is to the benefit of their community because it helps maintain resources and safety for them. Without this database in the system, they are at increased risk for unknown events. The personnel from the health departments regularly attended hemophilia board meetings, so that if there were complaints, somebody was there from the state level who could answer the questions and solved problems very quickly. One or two states ran into a few problems, but that was because of some unwise choices and not because they did not inform the community early and often. Those problems were also rectified, but it was not as smooth as in the states where they worked with the community in a more direct way.

The hemophilia registries are unusual in that hemophilia is a chronic condition, whereas most diseases reported to state health departments are infectious diseases. However, in the states where this surveillance was implemented, the health departments are addressing the issues of chronic diseases. They are more sympathetic to these approaches than health departments in some of the states where acute diseases are the only things that are reportable.

David Rothman: It is still a moderately scary precedent to have state legislatures pass these laws.

James Allen: It is obviously a very complex problem. It is not only a chronic condition, it is also a genetic condition, and that has many other implications.

CDC Surveillance for Unknown Pathogens

Scott Wetterhall

Surveillance has to be linked to public health action. The purpose of surveillance is to assess status, define priorities, evaluate programs, and stimulate research. The thesis that I am going to make, quite frankly, is that surveillance systems per se probably will not detect unknown pathogens or unknown etiologic agents. However, having ongoing surveillance systems provides a contact, an infrastructure, and a series of relationships such that detection can occur and a response can be mounted.

Some fundamentals are needed to do surveillance, such as an organized health care system, a system for classifying disease and injury, and measurement techniques. Surveillance has many different activities. For the purposes of this group, I would focus on triggering investigations or detecting epidemics as the best uses for public health surveillance.

You have heard about a number of different surveillance systems in the United States. Of these, the notifiable disease reporting system is the one that probably would serve as the basis for recognition of some sort of unknown pathogen or etiologic agent. This system exists in each of the 50 states and serves as a significant link between the Centers for Disease Control and Prevention (CDC) and the state health departments. There are other systems, and others are being developed—among them laboratory-based surveillance for antibiotic resistance patterns and hospital-based surveillance.

What is a notifiable disease? Some people don't realize this, but CDC cannot designate which diseases are notifiable. This authority is within the purview of either the state health board or the legislature of any given state. When AIDS became a notifiable disease in the 1980s, it was because laws or regulations were passed in each of those states. CDC works with the Council of State and Territorial Epidemiologists to determine what the notifiable diseases are. We currently have 51 diseases on our list. Diseases are added and deleted from this list. For instance, *Escherichia coli O157* has been added, as has antibiotic-resistant *Streptococcus pneumoniae*. Cases of these diseases are reported to CDC on a weekly basis.

You have heard a little bit about passive versus active surveillance. A passive system is one where physicians are required by regulation or law to report these diseases to local or state health departments. An active system, on the other hand, is one where reporting is initiated by a state health department.

The data are transmitted to CDC from state health departments electronically on a weekly basis and are published in the *Morbidity and Mortality Weekly Report*. For example, Figure 1 shows data tracking the decline in the number of cases or rate of malaria following World War II and subsequent rises primarily from returning veterans or foreign immigration. These data are available, and they are used to follow long-term trends.

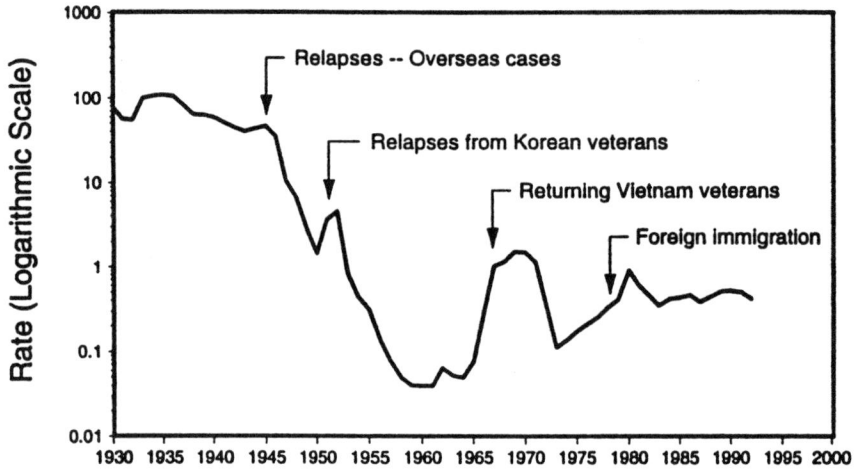

FIGURE 1 Reported cases of malaria per 100,000 population in the United States, 1930–1992.

How good are the data? Notifiable diseases carry with them regulations, fines, and various admonitions if a physician does not report a case of a particular notifiable disease. Yet we clearly know that there is a lot of underreporting. Table 7 presents data from Vermont comparing the number of patients hospitalized with notifiable diseases with the percentage of cases that are actually reported. Underreporting clearly is a problem, even though reporting is mandated by law.

TABLE 7 Evaluation of Notifiable Disease Reporting, Vermont, 1982–1983[52]

Disease	Hospital Cases	Percent Reported
Hepatitis	64	31
Aseptic meningitis	127	6
Bacterial meningitis	65	62
Gonorrhea	30	95
Pertussis	15	40
Salmonellosis	63	67

We have similar data from Washington, DC. They are about 10 years older, but the trends have basically been the same. There is tremendous underreporting of disease, except when new diseases occur, such as AIDS. The case reporting for AIDS has actually been fairly good for two reasons: it is a relatively new disease and it is an exotic disease. Also, a lot of money was put into surveillance for it.

There are several reasons for underreporting, and these are basically relevant to any surveillance system, particularly passive ones. There is often a lack of knowledge of reporting requirements, and there are negative attitudes toward reporting. There are misconceptions and even suspicion of the government and what it may be doing with this particular data.

What are the ways to improve the surveillance system? Make it simple. Systems are often far too complex for what they are intended to do. Provide frequent feedback, widen the net, get increasing sources of information, and conceivably, do active surveillance. There has been talk about active surveillance. The advantages are that you can identify all the cases, you get better-quality data, and some of the data may be useful in special circumstances. The disadvantages are that it is incredibly time-consuming and costly, and the additional data may not be worth the cost, except in special circumstances.

When new diseases emerge, we must have sufficiently simple, flexible, and acceptable systems already in place such that surveillance for these new pathogens or new disease entities can be incorporated into these systems quite readily.

Using as an example the current attention being directed toward emerging infections, CDC is undertaking efforts to improve its surveillance activities in

---

[52] Vogue, RL, SW Clark, S Kappel (1986). Evaluation of the state surveillance system using hospital discharge diagnosis, 1982–1983. *American Journal of Epidemiology, 123:* 197–198.

this arena. A number of major factors are contributing to the emergence of infectious diseases: human demographics and behavior, technology and industry, economic development and land use, international travel and commerce, microbial adaptation and change, and breakdown of public health measures. Increased population density and population encroachment, along with increases in international travel, are the same factors that would likely result in the introduction of some particular pathogen into the blood supply. The top seven emerging infectious diseases in 1993 were cryptosporidiosis, coccidioidomycosis, *E. coli* 0157:H7 disease, multidrug-resistant pneumococcal disease, vancomycin-resistant enterococcal infections, influenza A/Beijing/ 32/92 virus infections, and hantavirus infections.

I don't think these are necessarily ones that could be found in the blood supply, but the potential is always there for some emerging pathogen to find its way into the blood supply. These are new diseases or emerging diseases for which we need to form responses. Figure 2 provides data on the incidence of one of these, hantavirus. Hantavirus is a good example of the detection of a disease that wasn't previously notifiable. Emerging diseases are reported because people at the front line of public health (the public health nurses, physicians, primary care doctors, and medical examiners) notice an unusual syndrome and call up health officials. That is how you detect unusual or new diseases.

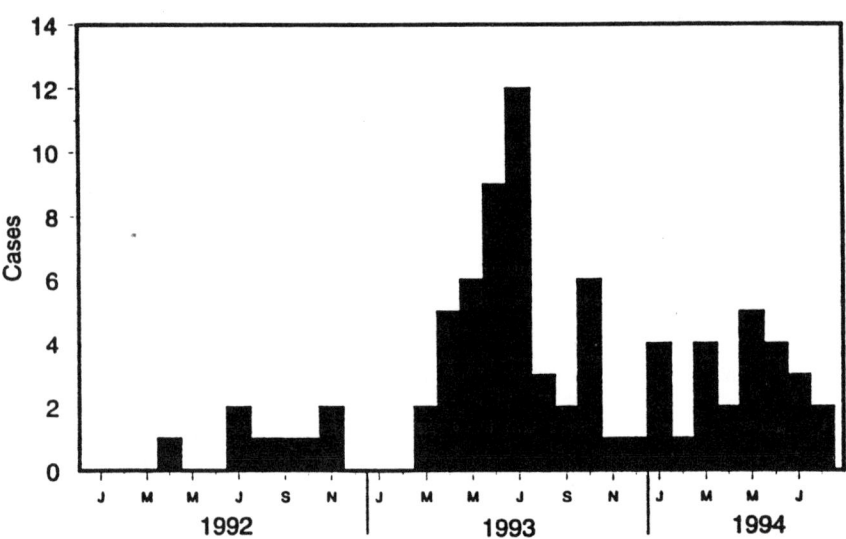

FIGURE 2 Reported cases of hantavirus pulmonary syndrome in the United States, January 1–August 31, 1994 (11 cases prior to 1992 not shown).

There have been several notable instances of outbreak detection going back to the 1970s. Legionnaires' disease was first detected when a Veterans Administration pathologist came in to the morgue over the weekend and found three or four elderly men who had died from pneumonia. He called up a friend at CDC to report that something was going on. You know the story of AIDS in terms of a physician noting a cluster of illnesses in a certain group as well as the increased medication use that was alluded to earlier. Hantavirus was reported by a medical examiner who called up a medical examiner at CDC. E. coli O157, which caused the famous multistate hamburger outbreak, was detected because a pediatric gastroenterologist noticed hemolytic-uremic syndrome in a young child. The salmonella-contaminated ice cream outbreak that began in Minnesota was detected by the use of state lab serotyping data. In the state lab in Minnesota where the serotyping takes place, they found an increased incidence in one of the serotypes, which resulted in an investigation and detection of a multistate outbreak.

Surveillance provides an infrastructure and relationships such that if something does happen, the person who notices something unusual can make the phone call. The calls can then be channeled to the appropriate persons. The CDC Epidemic Intelligence Service (EIS) is the active arm of CDC in terms of doing outbreak investigations. It was founded in 1951 because of concerns about biological and chemical warfare at the height of the Cold War and the Korean crisis. It is a training program that has graduated approximately 2,200 individuals from the program since its inception.

EIS officers are not the only ones who may detect outbreaks, but the training program serves as a very useful informal network, linked by a yearly directory, for making contacts with our colleagues as we identify new and unusual things. We are ingrained from day one as EIS officers with the steps of an outbreak investigation:

- establish existence of outbreak,
- verify diagnosis,
- define and identify cases, and
- characterize by time, person and place.

Then we must

- develop hypotheses,
- evaluate hypotheses,
- refine hypotheses and conduct additional lab and environmental studies, and
- implement control measures.

You learn these in a relatively rote way, but you find that they are useful for almost any situation, including the unknowns.

In the EIS network, 50 officers are currently have assignments in 26 state health departments. We have graduates in field epidemiology training programs in 19 countries. We also have a very active international visitor exchange program, such that often colleagues who are overseas detect things such as the Ebola virus outbreak in Zaire. They then give us a call and things begin to move along. It is an informal network, but it is a relatively effective one. It has worked well in the past in terms of identifying unknown pathogens.

Finally, we are researching the history of the notifiable disease surveillance system because it underscores a lot of interesting relationships between the federal government and states. Disease reporting is a state function, and Henry Baker, who was quite clairvoyant back in the beginning of this century, made this argument for collecting information on disease and health. "The only way to learn what diseases cause most sickness is to collect the statistics of sickness."[53] That serves as our foundation for identifying new and unusual pathogens. We continue to do that. Hopefully, we can do a better job at it.

DISCUSSION

Bernard Horowitz: You described a system that was put in place several years ago that is an extension of an older one for monitoring hemophiliacs. One of the arguments is to assess blood safety. By the very nature of the treatment of hemophilia A or hemophilia B patients, who are largely treated with concentrates which are highly purified and virally inactivated with solvent/detergent or other other techniques, it is not as complete a reflection of safety from viruses as, for instance, the use of other patient groups such as those with thalassemia. Are you aware of comparable systems for other groups of patients, or in what way are you using rare hemophiliacs to understand the infectivity of donated blood?

Bruce Evatt: I am not aware of other groups. I think that hemophilia patients are a unique group in that they are exposed to blood products from large numbers of donors. They are a sentinel group, but they now are also

---

[53]U.S. Public Health and Marine Hospital Service (1903). Transactions of the First Annual Conference of State and Territorial Health Officers with the United States Public Health and Marine Hospital Service. *Public Health Bulletin*, No. 11.

receiving more and more purified kinds of products. It is expected that their transfusion exposure will decrease in future years as they go to all recombinant products, except for the blood transfusions that they require.

James Allen: If money is to be made available for surveillance for transfusion-transmitted diseases or special issues of that sort, we need to be certain that we have a very strong local, state, and federal disease investigation system and general surveillance process rather than looking to build a superspecialized type of vehicle for something unknown. Instead, our general surveillance system must be very strong. I have very real concerns about the strength of that today.

III

New Ideas for Safety and Monitoring

Information Technology and Blood Safety

J. Michael Fitzmaurice

Assume there is a newly discovered virus in donor blood that is detectable by a test, and it is associated with a small number of people initially. You want to trace those who received the infected blood, and you may also want to trace those donors who were potentially exposed via their reported behavior. Maybe you can find that out through answers to their blood and interview questions. Do you have the information system to do it? What would it take to develop that capability?

I want to talk about what a computer-based patient record is, what a clinical decision support system is, what evidence there is that they work, what barriers stand in the way of the development of a computer-based patient record system, and then what is the applicability to a blood information system.

A computer-based patient record is just a collection of health data in electronic form and is part of the health information system of a physician or of a hospital. It could also be part of a health information system in a managed care organization or an insurance company. In electronic form that information is legible and available. When you ask for it, with the proper authority, you can get it, and if somebody else asks for it, they can get it at the same time. It is communicable, and you can search it.

It is also a powerful tool for organizing patient care data, improving patient care, and strengthening communication among health care providers. That may be one of its strongest points: retrieving medical knowledge that is applicable to that particular patient at the time you make a decision. The operating hypothesis is that computer-based patient record systems can improve both physician performance and patient outcomes of care.

The primary role for this collection of electronic data is to support the delivery of care to a particular patient. It brings the information to the physician, promotes communication, documents care, and records the reasoning behind the choices that are made. The secondary role of the computer-based patient record is to build a clinical data repository. All the data do not have to be linked together and located in one place, as long as you can find what you want and pull it in.

My agency, the Agency for Health Care Policy and Research (AHCPR), was created by Congress to determine what works in the community's practice of medicine. We know what works in the ideal setting of a clinical trial. In the community, patients behave differently and skill levels are not all the same. What are the differences? Why do we find so much variation across the country in procedures and in patient outcomes? These are important questions. The computer-based patient record is valuable for improving population-based care because you can query a large number of records and learn a great deal about the community factors that lead to those patient conditions and outcomes of care.

A clinical decision support system, utilizing computer-based patient records, is simply computer software that aids decision making by providing diagnostic suggestions, treatment suggestions, testing prompts, drug alerts for potential drug-drug or drug-food interactions, therapeutic protocols, and practice guidelines. AHCPR promotes the development of practice guidelines. We would love to be able to drop them into computerized patient record systems to find out what difference they make in the process of care and patient outcomes, and even to research and test patient care pathways.

A clinical decision support system requires a knowledge server, and that is simply a link between the patient and the information necessary for that patient's care. Normally, a physician is that link, but a physician using a mechanical instrument like a computer and a computerized record can do so much more and doesn't have to worry about forgetting.

What does a good clinical decision support system require? It requires a body of data about the patient that a physician considers important. It requires knowledge sources; if this, then that, and then that. How do I test for this; how do I test for that? Suppose I suspect a given diagnosis? In what order should I do the tests; do I do an X-ray, then an MRI (magnetic resonance image), then a CAT (computer-assisted tomography) scan, and then a PET (positron emission tomography) scan?

It requires a knowledge server that is the link between the computer-based patient record and the information source. You can describe the components of that knowledge server as medical logic modules, sentences that say, "If this is a female patient over 50 years old, and you don't find a Pap smear result in her record, then suggest that she get one. If you don't find a mammography result in her record, suggest that she get one. If the patient is 65 years of age, has asthma, and there is no evidence of an immunization for the most recent flu virus, suggest that the patient get one." It also needs a common nomenclature so that physicians talk the same language and can query the computerized knowledge base and can query the scientific literature using the same language, or else you need a good translator for that language.

These decision support systems improve patient care processes. In some cases they have measurably improved patient outcomes, but most of the studies that have looked at such systems are about improving patient care processes. For example, providing preventive care information to physicians and their patients improves compliance with immunizations. However, if you take the computer assist away, then immunization goes back down to previous levels. These systems also support diagnosis of high-risk patients, and of course, you often treat high-risk patients differently than you treat low-risk patients. The systems also help determine the sometimes toxic drug dose for obtaining the desired therapeutic levels. With these systems we can avoid having to look up in tables the many different patient factors and doing all of the extensive research necessary for a particular patient. If you haven't seen a patient like that for awhile, the computer can help you remember drug and test ordering.

In a clinical trial supported by AHCPR, the researcher had one set of physicians with regular computer screens for drug and test ordering and another set of physicians with special computer screens for drug and test ordering that were geared to question drug selection.[54] Both groups of physicians had screens and both groups did test ordering. Those with the special screens designed to question the choice of drug or test on the basis of the suspected diagnosis and medical knowledge found in the literature and to put cost savings suggestions up front wound up saving money and reducing lengths of stay. However, those physicians spent about 5.5 more minutes per patient per 10-hour shift. Thus, you have technology that improves the process of care, but costs the physician time. The physician does not get paid any more for the extra time. There must be some way to get the benefits down to the decision maker for taking the time to enter the information and query the system, thereby improving the care of the patient and the process of care.

Other studies, also funded by AHCPR and its predecessor, the National Center for Health Services Research, showed improved blood use through computer-based screening of orders, and that a computer-based patient interview elicited more HIV-related risk factors in the health histories of blood donors than one conducted by a staff member. These donors considered being queried by a computer to be more private, and they were more honest with their answers. We need to look at improving the sensitivity not only of the lab screening but of donor screening as well.

---

[54] Tierney, WM, ME Miller, JM Overhage, CJ McDonald (1993). Physician inpatient order writing on microcomputer workstations: Effects on resource utilization. *Journal of the American Medical Association, 269(3):* 379–383.

Clinical decision support systems also reduce malpractice threats. Massachusetts physicians have lower emergency room malpractice premiums if they use a particular system. The reason is not because the system results in better decisions, but because it produces better documentation. More court cases are lost because of a lack of documentation than because it is proven that someone made a bad decision.

If we are going to use these clinical decision support systems, what are some of the questions we need to answer? Most of the studies that I described were single-site studies in academic medical centers. We need more multiple-site tests of the same system. We need to know how much user performance is enhanced. We need to know how much patient outcomes are improved. In 10 randomized trials that were studied, only three of them measured patient outcomes. The others dealt with the process of care. You might assume that improving the process leads to improved patient outcomes, but that can be a big assumption—not necessarily a wrong assumption, but a big one. We need to know the costs of achieving these gains. Specifically, knowledge is needed about the costs of equipment, training, time, and energy spent convincing other peers to use a computer-based patient record system, as well as the costs of maintaining both a paper-based system and a computer-based system for a time so that people feel comfortable with the new system. We also need to investigate whether system-wide health care costs are contained, or we are just swapping one set of costs for another with no net gain.

We need to support an accessible medical knowledge base, and medicine is doing a good job of building that base. We also need to determine how strong a match of medical terms is needed, because we don't all talk the same language. How much do our words have to mean the same thing before we can communicate medical information upon which others are willing to act? How do we integrate clinical decision support systems into the environment and provide these systems with features that physicians will want, whether that involves communicating by typing, writing, speaking, or pushing a button.

The mechanism itself may be on your desktop, or maybe its a clipboard, or perhaps its hand held, or even at the bedside of the patient. Whatever it is, it must be flexible enough to improve the provider-patient relationship.

There is very little written in the scientific literature about how you best go about the implementation of these systems. What has led to success and what has led to failure? We know that physicians are reluctant to enter data; there is an uncertain effect on physician productivity and income. The confidentiality and privacy of physician's text notes are important to them, and there is also a variation in use of clinical decision support systems within a given hospital department by department. Those who are used to working with high-tech equipment are more willing to work with a computer-based patient record. Furthermore, there is insufficient information in the scientific literature about the factors that lead to the successful implementation of a clinical decision support system in hospitals and physicians' offices. One thing is certain: you will know they have arrived when managed care organizations begin using them extensively.

There are many extended uses of computer-based patient record data beyond the care of the specific patient. Among these are their use for research, quality assurance, patient care treatment paths, treatment strategies assessment and medical technologies assessment. Computer-based patient record data can provide information to a wide range of users for making many different choices, depending upon how they are aggregated and analyzed.

This patient care data should be

- uniformly defined,
- linked accurately
- collected together into databases, and
- held confidentially.

This is an ambitious vision. We don't as yet have widespread computer-based patient records. Some patient care data are normally computerized, such as lab records and radiology test reporting. Unfortunately, what happens is that the data are printed out of the auto analyzer onto paper and the paper is sent to the patient's floor, where two or three holes are punched in it and it is slapped into a paper medical record. We lose the advantage of computerization.

Today many decisions are based on data of inferior quality. Many decisions are made on the basis of claims data, not just Medicare claims data, which are the best in the world, but also private insurance company claims data. Decisions are being made on the basis of those large claims databases without sufficient clinical information. Clinical, medical record patient care data are becoming more valuable for decision making. For example, Kaiser Permanente has planned over the next 5 years to spend millions of dollars developing and implementing a computer-based patient record system. The Mayo Foundation is also developing a computer-based patient record system. To support the growing private sector use of computer-based patient records, AHCPR and the National Library of Medicine are funding eight test beds to test the commonality of nomenclature and how easy it is to exchange clinical information across different computer-based patient record systems.

What do you need to know if you are going to get involved in computer-based patient records? First, you need standards. You need definitions for signs, symptoms, and conditions of patients. That is, you need codes for the diagnoses of patients and procedures performed on patients, and they have to be used for more than just billing. You also need to define file contents. What data do you want to see to make a particular decision about whether to admit a patient to the hospital or to order another series of drug tests or order an X-ray? You need to define those data and be able to pull them up electronically for that decision.

Second, you need confidentiality and privacy protection for the patient care data. You need to define what is individually identifiable data, balance the benefits against the potential harm, and then specify what is a fair treatment of those data. In addition, someone has to be responsible for data quality assurance. When the data aren't accurate, somebody's head—not the patient's—has to roll.

Electronically stored records are essential, but the current environment is not especially receptive to their use. There are variations across states in health care privacy laws, regulations, and practices. Some states have "quill pen" laws, which means you have to sign in pen and ink for the medical record to be admissible as evidence in court. This rules out electronic signatures.

Third, standard unique identifiers for patients, health care providers, and payers must be developed. These are essential to obtain economies of scale in information technology.

Fourth, malpractice concerns must be addressed. Are you giving medical advice across borders when you are dealing with drug information? Do you need to be licensed in each state in which you are exchanging information? Who has legal jurisdiction in case there is an exchange of erroneous information and the patient is harmed?

Fifth, the security and integrity of your system must be ensured. You will have to deal with purposeful violations of privacy as well as accidental violations. You also have to deal with the accuracy of medical knowledge in clinical decision support systems and the accuracy of data transmissions. Who is to blame if important data get lost in the phone wire or an electronic switch or a faulty file server? Who is legally responsible for bad patient outcomes due to a flaw in a transmitted image or misreported medical knowledge?

We need better benefit/cost methodologies, but whose benefits and whose costs should be the focus of study? We have to assess the business risks, as well as the business benefits, because, after all, this is a business investment decision.

Once you have computerized patient records, can you pull the patient care data together into a regional health repository? How is it governed? Who owns the data? Who gets to use the data? Who sets the rules? Do the owners set it? Does the regulatory agency set it? Do you want all these data packed together in a centralized database or distributed? If distributed, every time you send a question out to be answered, do the data suppliers get to decide whether they want to answer your question or withhold the data?

What about the use of computerized patient records to register blood information? Let us assume that the purpose is to reduce the incidence of blood-borne disease by identifying and excluding bad blood using a computerized database. A second purpose could be to trace back to the source of the contaminated blood. Let us assume that you already have a computerized system in place. Then you identify the hurdles and how to overcome them.

We can assume that blood donors and recipients voluntarily report necessary personal information. What happens if they don't? Do you deny a transfusion to a patient who refuses to provide you with information? We can assume the patient consents to blood donation, collection of personal characteristics, linkage with other information, and disclosure, but to get that informed consent you may have to define exactly what disclosures you plan.

The use of the database has to be governed. Who does it? Government? The private sector? At a national level? At a local level? Again, you have to identify the hurdles and who is responsible for addressing them.

You have to have a disclosure policy. There is no federal privacy law that generally governs health data, except those related to AIDS and some other communicable diseases. By and large there is no federal law that protects the privacy of your own health data. You have to rely on your state and your health care provider.

Who determines the user authorization and that an inquiry is really from that authorized user? You need a system of inquiry, and you have to decide how you are going to respond to the inquiries: by computer, by telephone, in writing, or in person?

We have covered the database structure before when we talked about computer-based patient records, but do you have a database in each blood bank? Do you have a database nationally? You have to decide that. You need standards for this database, and you need to define the database content. What are you going to use to identify the person: Social Security number? Suppose the patient refuses? You say, "Well, then I will get the name, date of birth, sex, and mother's maiden name. That will give me 95 to 98 percent accuracy." But is that good enough?

You have to have some individual or some institution monitoring the data quality: confidentiality and privacy, what laws apply, who bears the legal responsibility for this, how secure the storage system is, and what protections is built into your system?

Then we get into system liability. Who is responsible? The caregiver is responsible for his or her own decisions, but when decisions are shared among several providers in separate states, how is responsibility determined? Who is responsible for the system liability? If you have information in the decision support system about contraindications, who is responsible for the integrity and accuracy of that information?

Finally, how do we overcome these barriers? Many people believe there should be a national privacy law that would set out appropriate uses of personally identifiable health data and specify the conditions under which they can be used. What are the penalties if somebody misuses these data? How much do they have to pay? How long do they have to spend in jail?

Should there be federal relief from liability due to system failure? Somebody ought to be liable for it. You might say, "Well, we can take care of that with federal no-fault compensation." Yes, but it comes out of the pockets of the taxpayers and creates undesirable incentives. Some things that could be useful to get a system off the ground may not be wise in the long term. There should be informed consent forms for both the donor and the patient. There should be a review of existing secured systems to know what kind of model to adopt for a secure blood bank registry system. And there should be a development of funding sources. Who benefits from this? If the public benefits, should there be a public payment for this? If it is solely a private benefit, then do you add the cost to the charge per unit of blood? Do major health insurers like the Health Care Financing Administration agree that a computerized system of blood records is needed, and will these insurers pay the additional charge? All of this should be pilot and market tested. You cannot just rush into it. You need to pilot test it in a couple of places, work out the kinks, look at the benefits, look at the costs, and then move ahead.

What is at stake is the potential to increase the value and security of our national blood and blood product system by using applications of health information technology. A greater knowledge of the barriers and hurdles will lead to better public and private solutions.

Strategies for Dealing with Potentially Infected Recipients

Ernest R. Simon

The basic premise underlying strategies for dealing with potentially infected recipients is that recipients may have a need, and certainly have the right, to know if they may have been infected. Clearly, with the right to know goes the right not to know. There is substantial evidence that, when asked, many recipients elect not to know if they may have been infected.

The second basic premise is that look-back is ineffective, inefficient, and certainly costly, more so for hospitals and physicians than for blood centers. Only a tiny portion of the time, effort, and cost of current look-back programs for human immunodeficiency virus (HIV) and human T-lymphotropic virus (HTLV) I/II yield productive results. With hepatitis C virus (HCV), the problems are magnified.

The issue is not look-back versus no look-back, but look-back versus something better than look-back. Look-back provides a cosmetic approach; I propose a substantive solution.

There are two situations, those dealing with future recipients (which I will discuss) and those dealing with prior recipients. For future recipients, a transfusion episode should be considered to consist of three distinct components: pretransfusion, the transfusion itself, and posttransfusion actions. Several weeks before the anticipated need, the prospective transfusion recipient should be provided with information regarding the benefits of transfusion, as well as risks and alternatives. In addition, the rationale for testing the potential recipient for infectious disease markers both prior to the transfusion and after the transfusion should be clearly explained. The patient should be told of possible personal benefits that testing might provide. Conditions may be revealed that modify the type of care that the patient should receive and may even help with diagnosis. It is important that the testing in no way interferes with the appropriate care that the patient may get on the basis of the results of the test. In addition, testing may possibly help identifiable partners of the patient avoid infection if the patient practices appropriate preventive behavior.

A second rationale deals with the possible benefit to hospital staff if they know of the presence of certain potential infectious agents in the patient. Despite the practice of universal precautions, such knowledge may provide additional safety to the hospital staff. And finally, pretransfusion testing may provide a baseline to assuage liability concerns.

It is clear that such viral marker testing is not necessarily limited to potential transfusion recipients. One can and should consider testing all surgical patients, or for that matter all patients, because the likelihood of the presence of infectious agents in patient populations is at least two orders of magnitude higher than it is in the volunteer donor population. Therefore, the yield of positive results from testing hospitalized patients is very much higher than is the yield from testing donors. Such viral marker testing is feasible for elective surgery. In the case of emergency surgery, a pretransfusion sample could be collected and held for subsequent testing as necessary.

The third phase of the transfusion episode takes place 6 to 12 months after the transfusion and completes the transfusion episode. At this time, the physician is reminded to contact the patient and/or the patient is reminded to contact the physician. The testing is repeated. If reactive results are obtained, confirmatory testing is done and the patient is counseled appropriately. This approach is analogous to other follow-ups, for example, in surgery, cancer cell therapy, and so forth.

For hepatitis B virus (HBV), HIV, HCV, and HTLV I/II, current testing may benefit the patient, a third party, or both. It is clear that both are benefited with HIV and HBV testing, but with HCV it is unclear whether a third party is benefited in addition to the patient. For HTLV I/II the benefits to the patient or third party are questionable. With current screening of the blood supply and pretransfusion testing of the patient, the incremental additional yield of positive results at 6 to 12 months posttransfusion would be expected to be very low.

The advantages over look-back are significant. Because posttransfusion follow-up is independent of the donor, it casts a wider net. It does not depend on a repeat donor who is now positive for the marker. It includes recipients of blood from one-time donors and repeat donors who have not returned or who have since been eliminated from the donor pool by surrogate tests performed prior to anti-HCV testing and donors who were subsequently disqualified without donating.

Furthermore, it reduces or eliminates unproductive administrative complexities including a tortuous and sometimes flawed records trail and interventions and follow-ups by blood centers, transfusion services, hospital records departments, and multiple physicians. It targets surviving recipients and avoids tracing deceased patients. It embraces future transmissible agents with ease and shortens the interval between putative transmission and detection. Finally, by acknowledging that zero risk for transfusion is not achievable now, it should be a powerful incentive to decrease the inappropriate use of blood components.

Implementation is simple. Informed choice, by which the patient is informed of possible unexpected outcomes, should precede the transfusion episode. On discharge the message can be reinforced and specific information regarding mechanisms for follow-up can be provided. The responsibility for follow-up could rest with the patient as it should, or it could be expanded by including the physician. If the patient is transfused and discharged alive, the hospital information system could trigger automatic reminders to the attending physician and/or the patient after 6 to 12 months.

An acceptable approach is essential. The specifics are not. By linking it to appropriate community and physician education with the active involvement of the U.S. Public Health Service, state and local health departments, medical and blood service organizations, blood centers, hospitals, manufacturers, and in particular the national media, routine posttransfusion follow-up becomes an extension of the HIV program recommended by the Presidential AIDS Commission and the American Hospital Association to its member hospitals. The message must emphasize that transfusion accounts for a small fraction of these diseases and that the focus on transfusion recipients is merely a part of our overall health strategy.

In summary, this approach to future recipients does not mean look-back versus no look-back, but look-back versus something better than look-back. The testing approach advocated is substantive. Look-back is cosmetic. A substantial yield of pretransfusion testing may be expected. The additional incremental yield of posttransfusion testing is expected to be very low given the sensitivity of currently used tests.

IV

Risk Tolerance

Beneficial Aspects of Surgical Transfusion

Richard K. Spence

Where do we find proof of benefit of surgical transfusion? That is a tough call. It is a routine procedure for donors to give blood and just as routine for physicians to obtain blood from a blood bank. Today's physician writes an order and the blood arrives thanks to the blood bankers. The practicing surgeon hardly gives it a thought.

Allogeneic blood is available for both elective and emergency surgery, which truly is an advantage of the use of allogeneic blood, because there is no burden on the patient. Use of autologous blood is not always an option. Patients must have enough time before surgery to donate the blood needed for the surgery. This becomes quite an issue in discussions about autologous predonation by patients, for example, with coronary artery disease. There is increasing evidence that heart surgeons, cardiologists, and others are moving patients to the operating rooms faster than they have before. Thus, we are seeing less and less autologous predonation in patients with coronary artery disease.

Although we surgeons take it for granted, where is the proof of benefit of transfusion? If we look through the literature for the prospective randomized controlled trial, we will not find it because we will not find an institutional review board (IRB) anywhere that will approve a trial of transfusion versus no transfusion in surgical patients. Therefore, analysis has to be based on retrospective data and anecdotal information. Another way to look for benefit is to see what harm might come from lack of a transfusion. These are the two approaches I took in trying to demonstrate benefit. Neither is proof positive, but both provide considerable evidence of benefit.

Before transfusion existed, preoperative preparation was prayer. Physicians wrote about the use of transfusion during the Middle Ages, but the use of transfusion really did not come into play until the technology emerged in the 1660s. The story of the history of transfusion follows on the heels of the description of the circulatory system by William Harvey. A friend of Harvey's, Sir Christopher Wren, described how to get access into the veins. He used a sharpened goose quill and an animal bladder and injected a variety of things into the vessels. The learned societies in England, France, and throughout the continent heard about this and said why not give blood to patients?

The first recorded transfusion was to Antoine Mauroy, a 34-year-old imbecile who had "escaped from his wife's control." He was transfused with several liters of calf's blood over 6 days, until his death.[55] Richard Lower did a transfusion at a similar time in England, but the French physicians Denis and Emmerez are the ones who get the credit for the first transfusion. Unfortunately, the issue of transfusion risk came into play with this first transfusion because Mauroy's widow sued for malpractice, blaming transfusion for her poor husband's death. As it turns out, she had poisoned the man with strychnine.

This experience, plus experience in England, was enough to make the national academies decide that transfusion was not such a good thing because the risks were so great. Thus, transfusion fell out of favor because it really did not seem to have a place in curing disease. Bear in mind that 17th century physicians thought the benefit of transfusion at the time was to restore mental capacity, to cure evil humors, and so forth. Transfusion was not looked at in a scientific way, such as we look at it today, until the early 1800s and James Blundell.

James Blundell was a physician-obstetrician in London who got tired of seeing his patients die of postpartum hemorrhage and wanted to do something about this. He was a very learned man who surely knew of the experiments conducted in the 1660s. He set about investigating this whole phenomenon in a scientific manner in the laboratory by instructing two postdoctoral students from Trinidad and Tobago to start transfusing animals. He began by giving lamb's blood to sheep, calves' blood to dogs, and so forth. He discovered quickly that you must stay within species in order to get some benefit from transfusion. With his London instrument makers he devised instruments to collect and administer blood with a syringe and a three-way stopcock. He used these devices in the clinical arena, salvaging blood from his bleeding patients and collecting blood from donors. There are some interesting treatises from this period concerning how to defibrinate blood to deal with clotting, including using birch twigs to stir the blood in order to impede clotting.

Blundell eventually began transfusing blood to his patients, and had about a 60 percent improvement in survival. In Blundell's work there was a change in the scientific approach to the use of transfusion. For the first time, Blundell was transfusing patients to treat blood volume loss and red cell loss, not to correct mental illness. His devices presaged modern blood equipment, and he

---

[55]Diamond, L (1980). A history of blood transfusion. In Weintrobe, MM (ed.), *Blood, Pure and Eloquent*. New York: Leonard & Co.

should perhaps be considered the father of modern transfusion medicine for his use of blood to treat anemia as a result of blood loss.

In 1883 Jennings published his summation of all of the works that had been written to that time concerning transfusion, which really was not very much. He looked at 243 cases of blood transfusion, and he again showed that two-thirds of these were successful in saving lives.[56] Most of these were for postpartum hemorrhage and the bulk of this material was Blundell's. In 1883, nothing was known about ABO and Rh blood groups. We now know that because of the distribution of blood types in the European/American populations (45 percent type O, 40 percent type A, 11 percent type B, and 4 percent type AB) the chances of inducing a serious reaction by transfusing without regard to ABO group are only about 35 in 100. Blundell, Jennings, and other transfusers of their time were fortunate. If the proportions of blood types in Europeans was different, we probably would not have seen transfusion advance as far as it did.

Bear in mind also that a risk-benefit analysis in this period of time could hardly have faulted Blundell for saving two-thirds more patients than he had before with the use of what was a highly risky procedure. He didn't know he was going to have problems with one-third of his patients, what we consider now a major risk—ABO incompatibility—but getting two-thirds of his patients to survive postpartum hemorrhage was recognized as an undeniable benefit of transfusion.

Early in this century scientific approaches to surgery continued to increase, promoting surgical procedures of a magnitude greater than we had seen before. This was initiated in part by anesthesia, which allowed patients to undergo larger and more complex surgical procedures. The surgical world had also heard from Rudolph Virchow, who had noticed that the ink from tattoos on the arms of his patients stopped in the lymph nodes in the armpit. He deduced that the lymph nodes must have a barrier effect, a function that might apply to cancer cells as well. He suggested that a way to treat patients with some specific forms of cancer might be to take out both the cancer and the lymph nodes. This marked the beginning of radical extirpative procedures: radical mastectomy, radical colon resections, and so forth. These procedures could not be done without the use of transfusion.

Transfusion medicine was still a relatively young science. In the early 1900s progress came mainly from the work of two pioneers: Alexis Carrell, who showed us how to do vascular anastomoses, and George Crile, Sr., who

---

[56]Jennings, C (1883). *Transfusion: Its History, Indications, and Modes of Application.* New York: Leonard & Co.

wrote *Hemorrhage and Transfusion*[57] in 1909 and again emphasized the necessity of replacing lost blood with transfused blood.

Transfusion soon became popular, and itinerant transfusionists, surgeons, and physicians who knew how to do this would travel around the country. It caught the public's attention. Despite great risks in this type of procedure, the benefits were clear to people at this time: preventing death from hemorrhage. As Bernheim said in his 1917 book *Blood Transfusion, Hemorrhage, and the Anemias*,[58] "Hundreds of people have been saved from premature death from hemorrhage." The literature contains many statements such as this, without any scientific basis for support such as a prospective or randomized trial. This was the perception of transfusion in general. Bernheim also pointed out an additional, indirect benefit of transfusion: operations could be made less hazardous with transfusion. Not only were they made less hazardous, but many were also made possible for the first time.

Before blood banks, transfusion required 2 patients and a surgical procedure. The ability to store blood temporarily in a "blood bank" led to further advances. Being able to take the blood out of the patient and separate it temporarily and then infuse it made it possible to transfuse more patients more easily.

Some of the surgical procedures that Bernheim foresaw as becoming possible are listed below. This list is by no means complete, but these are the kinds of things that would not be done today if it were not for transfusion. Even though for a percentage of patients some of these surgical procedures can be done without transfusion, that is only because of the skill and technology of people who have been working in this field for a number of years with blood close at hand.

- Transplantation. Renal, cardiac, and particularly liver transplants could not have been done without transfusion.
- Burn excision. Blood loss is very high in burn excision, and the techniques we have learned now rely on and depend on transfusion.
- Radical cancer surgery. The extirpative kinds of procedures such as mastectomies, pancreatoduodenectomies with the Whipple procedure, rectal excisions, hepatic resections, and radical prostatectomies all require transfusion.
- Other surgery made possible by transfusion: cardiac surgery, valve replacement, coronary artery bypass grafts, and vascular procedures of all sorts.

---

[57]Crile, G Sr. (1909). *Hemorrhage and Transfusion; An Experimental and Clinical Research.* New York and London: D. Appleton and Co.

[58]Bernheim, BM (1917). *Blood Transfusion, Hemorrhage, and the Anemias.* Philadelphia and London: Lippincott.

In the late 1960s and 1970s, it was routine to type and cross-match 25 to 26 units of blood in preparation for surgery. This is no longer done, but without the ability to transfuse large amounts of blood we would not have seen cardiac surgery advance to where it is today.

Since the mid-1980s we have seen about a quarter of a million coronary artery bypass grafts done each year. The patients who receive blood in this group represent about 10 percent of all blood recipients. At Cooper Hospital-University Medical Center in Camden, New Jersey, about 10 to 15 percent of overall red cell recipients in 1994 were coronary artery bypass recipients. This is a 550-bed university tertiary-care hospital where about 300 to 400 coronary bypass procedures are done per year, so there is a significant number of patients who are transfused in conjunction with cardiac surgery.

The Sanguis study has looked at 43 hospitals in Europe with more than 7,000 patients since about 1990. Some reports are starting to come out from the information gathered. Of all the patients studied and the number of procedures they looked at, 87.7 percent of coronary bypass patients were transfused.[59] Thus, transfusion is still a major part of coronary bypass surgery. More than 80 percent of vascular surgery patients were transfused. That includes both autologous and allogeneic blood, but even considering only allogeneic or banked volunteer donor blood, the numbers are still in the 35 to 50 percent range. Although we are doing better in terms of using autologous blood, we still need allogeneic blood to make these kinds of procedures possible.

The discussion to this point has been primarily about red cell transfusion, but therapy with platelets and plasma derivatives is an issue here as well. In 1991 it was reported that platelets are a major part of treatment of coagulopathies associated with cardiopulmonary bypass surgery, particularly in the pediatric age group. Platelets play a major role in coronary surgery as well. When we look at a listing of the primary users of platelets in hospitals we find that the coronary bypass patients are generally in the top one or two positions.

Other areas of medicine that would not be possible today without transfusion include level I trauma centers. Orthopedic surgical cases also would be impossible without transfusion. The Sanguis study has shown that 80 to 81 percent of all total hip patients are transfused. Likewise, surgery on patients with coagulopathies would be impossible. Operations such as simple inguinal hernia repair on a patient with hemophilia would not be done without anti-hemophilic factor derived from plasma. Even without surgery, patients

---

[59]Group TSS (1994). Use of blood products for elective surgery in 43 European hospitals. *Transfusion Medicine, 4:* 251–268.

with hemophilia and the inherent coagulopathies would all die at young ages because we would not have the plasma derivatives with which to treat them.

Another way to look at this is to ask what kind of surgery would we do without transfusion? It comes down to surgery that does not invade a body cavity. We can generally do laparoscopic surgery without transfusion, laparoscopic cholecystectomies for example. But surprisingly, the Sanguis Study found that about 15 to 20 percent of those patients are transfused as well. Without the backup of transfusion we would not be doing surgery as we know it today. It cannot be quantified in the same way that risk can with a number like 1 in 250,000, but the benefit is still clear.

In summary we can see the progression in surgical red cell transfusion:

• Treat shock. After early attempts to cure any and all diseases with transfusion, Blundell, and later Jennings, shifted attention to treating hemorrhage. In the 1900s Crile talked about hemorrhage and transfusion in shock. Blood was used for a long time to restore volume. The experience with World War I, and on into World War II, when blood became more available, supports this.

• Promote well being. Once blood became more and more available and the risks were still fairly minimal, transfusion was done for a lot of reasons that perhaps are not physiologically appropriate, such as perking up patients and putting a little pink in their cheeks. Fortunately, we have gotten away from a lot of that.

• Allow surgery. First and foremost, transfusion's benefit for surgery has been to save lives, by allowing interventions that would otherwise not be possible.

• Correct coagulopathy. The primary reason we should use red cell transfusion now is to improve oxygen delivery.

All of the foregoing has been focused on life-saving interventions. Another way to look at benefit is, as mentioned at the outset, to look at what kind of harm we see or what kind of damage is done if patients are not transfused when appropriate. To find that information we must look at the studies of patients who refuse transfusions, primarily the Jehovah's Witnesses. There are only a few studies, but there are survivors with hemoglobin (Hgb) levels as low as 3 to 5 g/dl. Some hemodilution studies also provide us information about the harm thta can occur if we do not transfuse. Jeff Carson and I did some work in early 1988 with a series of 125 surgical Jehovah's Witness patients.[60] This work showed that there were multiple comorbid

---

[60]Carson, JL, RK Spence, RM Poses, G Bonavita (1988). Severity of anemia and operative mortality and morbidity. *Lancet, ii:* 727–729.

factors that increased mortality in the Jehovah's Witness as hemoglobin level declined (e.g., cardiopulmonary disease), but mortality clearly was inversely related to preoperative hemoglobin level. We also looked at a subset of these patients who underwent elective surgical procedures.[61] The difference in mortality associated with low preoperative hemoglobin is small but significant: 5 percent for patients with preop Hgb between 6 and 10 g/dl versus 3.2 percent for those with pre-operative Hgb > 10 g/dl. A difference of only 1.8 percent may not seem like a lot, but if one considers the 2 to 3 percent mortality now viewed as acceptable in a quarter million coronary bypass patients, then this small difference represents both a large number of patients and a doubling of the operative risk.

Jeffrey Carson and I have now studied 528 patients: 206 Jehovah's Witnesses, and 322 who are not, looking at mortality and hemoglobin levels. Although analysis of this information is just beginning, it appears that in the 19 percent of these patients who were transfused we may be able to demonstrate for the first time that transfusion is a positive benefit in terms of increasing survival or preventing mortality. In brief, we begin to see a significant difference in mortality at a Hgb level of 7 g/dl and below. That is, patients who can be transfused—non-Jehovah's Witnesses who got down to 7 g/dl and were transfused—had lower mortalities than the comparable Jehovah's Witness patients who were not transfused.

We have also learned a lot from the laboratory and from the intensive care units about specific patient needs and some things that can happen if we do not transfuse. We have a much better idea about how the body adapts to anemia and the multiple factors that influence this: severity of anemia, competency of the cardiovascular and respiratory systems, oxygen requirements of the individual, and duration of the anemia.

The competency of the cardiovascular system seems to be the main determinant of how patients respond and compensate for surgical anemia. Patients maintain oxygen delivery when they are anemic by increasing cardiac output, simplistically, by increasing either heart rate or stroke volume. The first requirement for this is a healthy heart. The heart provides these compensatory changes by dilating coronary arteries. This response clearly is limited in the presence of coronary artery disease.

Two recent studies have shown an increased incidence of cardiac abnormalities in vascular surgery patients with postoperative Hgb levels below

---

[61] Spence, RK, JA Carson, R Poses, S McCoy, M Pello, J Alexander, J Popovich, E Norcross, RC Camishion (1990). Elective surgery without transfusion: influence of preoperative hemoglobin level and blood loss on mortality. *American Journal of Surgery, 159(3):* 320–324.

10 g/dl.[62] These two studies sounded the warning bell about *under*transfusion. If we look for more of this evidence, we would find that morbidity and mortality does increase in patients whose Hgb level is below 10 g/dl, particularly if they have coronary or pulmonary disease.

Jefferey Carson has been looking at a database of 1,400 or 1,500 nontransfused Jehovah's Witness patients. He has developed some preliminary information that seems to show that if we look at preoperative hemoglobin level, going from 14 g/dl down to 2 g/dl and look separately at patients with and without cardiopulmonary disease, mortality clearly increases in the presence of cardiopulmonary disease when preoperative hemoglobin is less than 10 g/dl. One can assume from this that transfusion should have a beneficial effect in these patients.

Gerson Greenburg has done some seminal work in this area and is beginning to move us toward what you might term a physiologic transfusion trigger of 12 ml of oxygen per minute per kg.[63] He has shown in a number of settings that this seems to be the lower limit for the heart. Below this level the heart muscle starts to deteriorate or convert to anaerobic metabolism. Thus, we are beginning to see the possibility of a more exact determination of when to employ transfusion. There are clear limits to cardiac response in anemia, but we may be able to override these with transfusion.

Let me digress for just a minute to talk about trauma. We have known for some time with a number of animal studies that there is a finite limit to the amount of volume that can be replaced with asanguinous fluids. We can quantify that to some extent in trauma. It is now well known that one of the things that we need to do in trauma is to move quickly; the golden hour concept that Donald Trunkey has popularized has led to the establishment of level I trauma centers around the country.

The trauma center in Camden is a fairly busy one, with about 1,800 patients a year. That means admitting a seriously injured patient every 5 hours throughout the year. In 1994, 26 percent of all red cells and components went to trauma patients; thus, the trauma patients are prime users of blood in the hospital. It is that transfused blood which gets these patients into the hospital, into the operating room, and treated within that golden hour. Hemorrhage may be classified into four levels by amount of blood lost. When we reach class three hemorrhage, the standard for fluid replacement is crystalloid and blood.

---

[62]Nelson, AH, LA Fleisher, SH Rosenbaum (1993). Relationship between postoperative anemia and cardiac morbidity in high-risk vascular patients in the intensive care unit. *Critical Care Medicine, 21(6):*860–866. Christopherson, R, S Frank, E Norris, et al. (1991). Low postoperative hematocrit is associated with cardiac ischemia in high-risk patients (abstract). *Anesthesiology, 75(3A):* A100.

[63]Greenburg, A (1988). Indications for transfusion. *Scientific American Medicine, 3:* 1–16.

If blood is not replaced at this point we start to see anaerobic metabolism, tissue loss, and patient death. The benefit is pretty clear in trauma, as transfusions allow us to move patients forward faster and also allow us to do the surgery needed to save lives.

One last area of medicine where transfusion is prominent is the anemia thatresults from chronic diseases, chronic infections, inflammations, malignancies, and so forth. It is facile to say that one should just correct the underlying disease that causes the anemia, but in fact this is not always that easy to do. Transfusion thus becomes an important part of treatment in these patients when they require surgery.

In conclusion, let me summarize the evidence for the beneficial effects of transfusion. There is some evidence that there would be limitations to surgery without transfusion. Many of the things we consider commonplace in surgery now would not be done without transfusion. There is some evidence in studies of Jehovah's Witnesses associating increased morbidity and mortality with lower hemoglobin levels, and we are beginning to get evidence that transfusion can turn that around. There is evidence for red cell-related limits of cardiac compensation, and we are beginning to acquire more solid physiologic findings about those limits that will help us to determine in the future just what we can do and what the transfusion intervention will provide. Finally, there are known tolerable limits to red cell loss from hemorrhage.

I would close by urging you to remember, as you contemplate the risks and benefits of transfusion, that all solutions create new problems; good solutions are those that introduce problems more manageable than those they replace.

Trade-off of the Risk of Hepatitis and the Benefit of Clotting Factor Concentrates in the 1970s and 1980s

M. Elaine Eyster

I want to discuss the trade off of the risks of hepatitis and the benefits of clotting factor concentrates in the pre- and post-AIDS era for persons with hemophilia. I do this as a hemophilia treater who has been caring for a large number of patients with hemophilia since about 1973 and as one of many involved with a large study on persons with hemophilia. That study, which has now become known as the Multicenter Hemophilia Cohort Study, began in September 1982 and was a collaborative research effort with James Goedert from the Viral Epidemiology Branch of the National Cancer Institute. The study currently involves hemophiliacs from 16 centers in the United States and Europe.

The acceptance of hepatitis risk by physicians and persons with hemophilia must be considered in the context of the prevalence of hepatitis B virus (HBV) markers, the apparent benign and nonprogressive course of non-A, non-B hepatitis, and the benefits of clotting factor concentrates as we knew them in the pre-AIDS era.

Following the introduction of pooled plasma fractions in the late 1960s, a 30 percent incidence of acute hepatitis was reported in first-time recipients of Factor VIII concentrate.[64] During the middle to late 1970s high rates of liver function abnormalities accompanied by very high rates of peripheral blood markers for HBV were reported in those patients who were repeatedly exposed to both cryoprecipitates and clotting factor concentrates. However, the vast majority of those with hepatitis remained asymptomatic, and the histologies of the few who underwent liver biopsies were consistent with non-A, non-B hepatitis, which appeared to be benign and nonprogressive.

---

[64]Kasper, CK and SA Kipnis (1972). Hepatitis and clotting factor concentrates. *Journal of the American Medical Association, 221:* 510.

By the early 1980s it was recognized that almost all frequent users of clotting factor concentrates had markers for hepatitis B. However, 90 to 95 percent had antibodies that conferred protective immunity and only 5 to 10 percent were chronic carriers of hepatitis B surface antigen, and for the most part these people appeared healthy. Serious liver disease and fatalities were rare, and by 1983 a hepatitis B vaccine was licensed. Little attention was paid to the persistently elevated or fluctuating transaminase values that were so characteristic of non-A, non-B hepatitis because the symptoms were mild and self-limiting and because many individuals suffered no clinical illness whatsoever.

Over the 5-year period from about 1977 to 1982, there was mounting evidence of chronic hepatitis in the majority of multitransfused hemophiliacs who had elevated transaminase levels. However, cirrhosis was infrequent, and there was still no evidence by 1982 (when the first cases of AIDS were reported in persons with hemophilia) that chronic liver disease increased morbidity or mortality. Furthermore, the first prospective study, in 1982, which included 11 hemophiliacs who were followed for 6 years with liver biopsies every 3 years, concluded that chronic liver disease was nonprogressive in those who had no intrahepatic hepatitis B markers.[65] It was not until 1985, when the epidemic of HIV infections in persons with hemophilia was nearly over, that the serious and the progressive nature of hemophiliac liver disease presumably due to non-A, non-B was suspected. It was not until 1989, after 10 years of intense research, that the non-A, non-B agent was finally identified as hepatitis C.

Today epidemiologic, serologic, virologic, clinical, and histologic studies strongly implicate hepatitis C as the major cause of chronic liver disease among persons with hemophilia. Those persons who received clotting factor concentrates during the 1970s and the 1980s, before the advent of viral inactivation procedures, were almost universally infected, and those who received repeated infusions of cryoprecipitate also had a high rate of infection. The vast majority of those who were infected remained chronically infected.

We know now from retrospective studies of stored sera that most concentrate recipients became infected with hepatitis C at the time of their first exposure to clotting factor concentrates which were made from pools of blood from 20,000 or more donors. Furthermore, we know the risk of hepatitis C infection to the recipients of these concentrates persisted until more effective viral inactivation procedures were developed in the late 1980s, and until donor screening tests for hepatitis C were implemented in 1990.

---

[65]Mannuci, PM, M Colombo, M Rizzetto (1982). Nonprogressive course of non-A, non-B chronic hepatitis in multitransfused hemophiliacs. *Blood, 60:* 655–658.

To understand why physicians and patients alike accepted this risk of hepatitis B and non-A, non-B hepatitis during the 1970s and early 1980s, we need to review the benefits of clotting factor concentrates and the risk of serious or fatal bleeding in the absence of clotting factor replacement therapy. The availability of these freeze-dried clotting factor concentrates radically changed the treatment of persons with severe hemophilia. They brought about dramatic improvements in the lifestyles and longevity of these individuals. Let me give you two examples to illustrate this.

The first is that of a man in his 40s who grew up without the benefits of clotting factor concentrates. He had severe Factor IX deficiency, and he was treated only with fresh frozen plasma during his youth. He spent most of his adult life in a wheelchair. I never saw this man out of a wheelchair for the 10 years that I cared for him.

The second is a youngster with severe Factor VIII deficiency who was treated with clotting factor concentrates from an early age as part of a home infusion program. He grew up with the philosophy, "When in doubt, treat to prevent irreparable joint damage and other complications from persistent bleeding into soft tissues." His mother was taught to infuse him at home when he was about 5 years old, and as he approached adolescence he was taught to infuse himself at the first sign of any bleeding. Early treatment with lyophilized concentrates that could be conveniently stored and carried almost anywhere enabled him to establish his independence as a teenager and to take part in most activities, including physical education classes, without disruption. This would not have been possible if he had had to rely on cryoprecipitates that needed to be stored in a home freezer and pooled before reconstitution.

In a study by the Orthopedic Hospital in Los Angeles from 1963 to 1965, before the availability of concentrates or cryoprecipitates, hemophilic elementary schoolboys missed an average of 35 schooldays per year, compared with an average of 11 days for their peers. In secondary schools, hemophilic adolescents missed six times as many days as other boys.[66]

In 1971, during an era when most patients were treated with single-donor products such as cryoprecipitates or fresh frozen plasma, a study by the National Heart, Lung and Blood Institute (NHLBI) found that only one-fourth of all hemophiliacs ages 6 to 24 were in school. Of those who were not in school, 30 percent were absent because of poor health.[67] In 1970, the median age of hemophiliacs in the United States was 11.5 years, compared with a median age of 26.8 years for the U.S. male population at that time. By 1982, the median age was 20 years compared with a median age of 29.3 years for

---

[66]Petit, CR and HG Klein (1976). *Hemophilia, Hemophiliacs and the Health Care Delivery System.* DHEW Publication No. (NIH) 76-871. Washington D.C.: Government Printing Office.
[67]*Ibid.*

U.S. males. This decrease in the overall mortality rate for persons with hemophilia was coincident with the widespread use of clotting factor concentrates, which replaced cryoprecipitate as the standard of care in the 1970s. By 1982, three-fourths of the nation's hemophiliacs were being treated with lyophilized concentrates. More than one-half of these received treatment in home settings, compared with only one-tenth in 1970.

With the transition to home care and early treatment with clotting factor concentrates, hospitalizations and visits to emergency rooms declined, and patients and their families experienced freedom from hospital dependency. In a study from the Hemophilia Center of Rhode Island, within 3 years after the implementation of a home therapy program the number of inpatient hospital days per year among persons with severe hemophilia decreased from 13 to 3.5 days, and the number of visits to the emergency room and clinic fell from 17 to 2.4 days per year.[68] Deaths attributed to hemorrhage, particularly central nervous system (CNS) bleeding, declined 33 percent between 1968 and 1979. However, in 1982, hemorrhage remained the most important cause of death among hemophiliacs, accounting for 40 percent of deaths and a 30 percent increase in mortality compared with that for all U.S. males.[69] Therefore, patients were encouraged to continue treatments and to do so as early as possible. Then AIDS struck and everything changed. By the time we recognized the problem, the majority of persons with severe hemophilia were already infected. Of those frequently treated hemophiliacs who became infected by contaminated concentrates, we learned retrospectively that more than one-half had already been infected by January 1983.[70]

We heard earlier about the value of repositories for sera. The reason that the retrospective studies of hemophiliacs were possible was because of sera which were collected for purposes other than surveillance. At our institution they were collected as part of a cooperative study sponsored by NHLBI in the mid-1970s having to do with the development of inhibitors in persons with Factor VIII deficiency. However, because of these kinds of repositories, a retrospective analysis could be done to document seroincidence as well as seroprevalence.

---

[68]Smith, PS, NC Keyes, EN Forman (1982). Socioeconomic evaluation of a state-funded comprehensive hemophilia care program. *New England Journal of Medicine, 306:* 575–579.

[69]Johnson, RE, DN Lawrence, BL Evatt, et al. (1985). Acquired immunodeficiency syndrome among patients attending hemophilia treatment centers and mortality experience of hemophiliacs in the United States. *American Journal of Epidemiology, 121:* 797–810.

[70]Kroner, BL, PS Rosenberg, LM Aledort, et al. (1994). HIV-1 infection incidence among persons with hemophilia in the United States and Western Europe, 1978–1990. *Journal of Acquired Immunodeficiency Syndrome, 7:* 279–286.

By January 1983, when the *New York Times* published its first report of a potential threat to the blood supply, 80 to 90 percent of persons with hemophilia who became infected from contaminated concentrates had already been infected. By January 1984, nearly 95 percent had been infected. Remember that in 1983 the AIDS incidence was only 0.6 percent in persons with hemophilia.

In the aftermath of the epidemic for persons with hemophilia, clotting factor concentrates have undergone stringent virucidal treatments and are believed to be "safe" once again. How safe are they? We know that the lipid-enveloped viruses are inactivated by treatment with solvent detergent or heat, but the nonenveloped viruses such as B19 parvovirus and hepatitis A virus are much more resistant. Fortunately, parvovirus infections are usually mild or asymptomatic in persons with hemophilia. Hepatitis A due to transfusions is rare, and we now have a vaccine to prevent hepatitis A. However, what about the potential for transmission of Creutzfeldt-Jakob disease (CJD) or some other slow-acting viral agent? What about the potential for blood-borne transmission of some deadly virus that is as yet unknown?

Many might say that these risks are no longer an issue for most persons with hemophilia because recombinant Factor VIII is now licensed and is widely available and recombinant Factor IX concentrate is now in clinical trials. However, what about the potential for contamination by an animal virus in the cell lines that are used to produce the recombinant factors? What about the potential for contamination of the fetal calf serum in which the cell lines are grown with a prion such as the one that is supposed to cause CJD? What about the potential for ill effects from trace amounts of mouse proteins from the monoclonal antibodies that are used to purify these factors? What about the potential for transmission of human viruses by the albumin which is still used as a stabilizer in these products? These theoretical risks are not meant to scare patients, nor are they meant to deter them from using the products upon which they depend for their lives, their livelihoods, and their independence. We all know that many steps are incorporated into the process of manufacturing recombinant Factor VIII which should eliminate all known infectious agents that might contaminate the end product, but just how safe are clotting factor concentrates today?

Today the benefits of clotting factor concentrates are as obvious as they were in 1982. Today the apparent risks are so low that they are largely unmeasurable, but except for hepatitis B and hepatitis non-A, non-B, they were unmeasurable in 1982. Now, as then, the alternative of no treatment is just as unacceptable to everyone concerned. Today, in spite of the potential risks, clotting factor concentrates remain the standard of care for the treatment of persons with severe hemophilia.

DISCUSSION

Harold Sox: Why did it take so long for hepatitis C to become recognized as something to be avoided rather than something to be put up with?

Elaine Eyster: Those of us who were caring for persons with hemophilia recognized it. For a majority of them transaminase levels were measured from time to time. Sometimes they would be abnormal. Sometimes they would be normal. Some persisted in having abnormal transaminase levels, but we noticed this year after year, and the patients were well. They had no clinical illness that anyone could detect, and the hemophilia-related bleeding problems were so overwhelming that it didn't seem appropriate to focus an undue amount of attention on these laboratory abnormalities. At the same time research was going on, but we really couldn't do much about the problem until we had a diagnostic test to identify the agent that was causing the elevated transaminase levels.

By 1990, a huge amount had been learned about this, and we are just now beginning to learn about the natural history of hepatitis C. If you talk to many persons with hemophilia who received clotting factor concentrates during that era, you will find that it would have been intolerable to them to think about not having these products to provide them with the kind of life that was worthwhile for them. Everyone relied on these concentrates at the time in order to make it possible for these persons to lead as normal a life as possible and to prevent risks from bleeding, particularly CNS hemorrhage, which was then and is still the major cause of death in HIV-negative persons with hemophilia.

Paul Russell: Why is it necessary to have such large pools? I know the risk is very much dependent on the size of the pool. Is there some scientific reason for it, or is it a practical matter of production?

Elaine Eyster: All I know is that the pools can range anywhere from a few thousand, say, perhaps 5,000 (the average was about 20,000), and subsequently I have heard reports of as many as 50,000 donors.

Comment from the audience: The Food and Drug Administration requires a minimum of at least 1000 different donors in pools from which gamma globulin is prepared, so as to include a wide variety of antibodies in the product. FDA standards for lot-to-lot consistency are also easier to meet with increasing numbers of donors in each lot, since the effects of anomolous donations are diluted. More to the point, pool size reductions do not effectively reduce risk for patients who require lifelong treatment.

Bernard Horowitz: If the issue is non-A, non-B hepatitis or hepatitis C, you have to take into account the fact that the underlying risk at that time for just blood from a single donor was something close to 1 percent. Why didn't you as a treater or any of the treaters do something to avoid exposure to hepatitis C? It is very easy to calculate that even going to a single-donor product would not have helped. With respect to the pool size, it certainly would not have helped if it is not going to even help at a single-donor level. It is just not relevant to hepatitis C at that time. Did you see any difference in hepatitis C transmission rates among the users of cryoprecipitate who would use 100, 300, or 1,000 units, compared with those among the users of concentrates?

Elaine Eyster: No. Once a person with severe hemophilia took the amount of cryoprecipitate that it took to treat his disease, there was virtually no difference in the incidence of hepatitis C, because he would soon be taking 1,000 units of cryoprecipitate derived from 1,000 different donors.

Henrik Bendixen: I can understand why hepatitis was tolerated in the hemophilia population because the trade-off was so outstanding. It is more difficult to understand why it was tolerated for so long in patients who received transfusions for, for example, surgical operations, in whom the incidence of hepatitis was considerable. And although mortality was not known to be a great problem, morbidity certainly was. That morbidity alone in the general population should have made us a little bit more intolerant than we were.

Harvey Klein: It was not widely appreciated until Harvey Alter's longitudinal study over a 20-year period that there was significant morbidity, let alone mortality. There was no excess liver-related deaths in transfused individuals, and the pathologists kept saying, "Where is all the cryptogenic cirrhosis that we are supposed to be seeing at autopsy in recipients of blood?" The answer was that it wasn't being seen. It took important, expensive longitudinal studies, primarily by an individual who stayed at the same institution for about 30 years and followed both the patients and the recipients, to demonstrate scientifically that not only was it present but that it was of clinical import.

Lew Barker: I find this word "tolerate" a little bit strange. We tolerate graft-versus-host disease in people who have transplants. People who work in hepatitis were always looking for tests so that they could do something about it. When there were tests that were nonspecific, they were extensively evaluated. There were meetings on the question of the extent of pathogenesis. Until specific tests were available, the situation was very murky, and the solutions were not at hand.

Examples of Risks That We Tolerate

Harvey G. Klein

What risks do we tolerate and what risks don't we tolerate? The *Leishmania tropica* paradigm is illustrative. During Operation Desert Storm we sent one-half million men and women to the Persian Gulf and from that half million 31 service personnel later developed symptoms that were associated with infection by *L. tropica*.[71] *L. tropica* was not transmitted by blood transfusion. However, a related parasite, *Leishmania donovani*, has a parasitemic phase. While there is a case in the literature of a transmission by a blood transfusion, clearly this is not a major public health problem. However, in the aftermath of AIDS and out of concern for the potential transmission of leishmaniasis, the Armed Forces made the decision to defer one-half million potentially eligible blood donors for a year. There was great discussion about this decision at the time. The outcome tells us something about the general tolerance for infectious diseases or potentially infectious diseases transmitted by the blood supply.

We have known for many years that transmission of bacterial infections by whole blood and by platelets occurs. Perhaps 1 in 1,000,000 infected red blood cell units transfused causes significant clinical outcomes because of bacterial contamination. As many as 1 in 2,500 platelet concentrates may transmit bacteria that are clinically important. But this doesn't seem to have raised the public ire. We tolerate this because there is no secondary transmission, because these are generally treatable infections if discovered in time, and because the fatality rate isn't appreciable or appreciated except for what we report to the Food and Drug Administration (FDA). "Tolerate" does not, however, imply acceptance or approval.

There was considerable excitement a couple of years ago about one of these organisms, *Yersinia enterocolitia*. *Y. enterocolitia* is a gram-negative aerobic rod that produces endotoxin, requires iron and carbohydrate for growth,

---

[71]Persian Gulf Veterans Coordinating Board (1995). Unexplained illnesses among Desert Storm veterans. *Archives of Internal Medicine, 155:* 262–268.

grows well at 4°C, and infects red blood cells stored at that temperature. Prior to 1987, only six cases of transfusion-related transmission had been reported. Then ten cases and seven deaths associated with red cell transfusions were reported in the United States between 1987 and 1993. All of the recipients became symptomatic during the transfusion, but all the donors were well at the time. However, when careful epidemiologic studies were performed by the Centers for Disease Control, five of the nine donors had had gastroenteritis within 4 weeks of donation and all of the infected units had been stored for more than 25 days. The suggestion was made that blood banks could deal with this issue by either using screening histories or shortening the storage interval of blood. When you try to screen a large population of donors for gastroenteritis, you will find a lot of gastroenteritis within the last 2 weeks of donation. Questions about gastroenteritis didn't seem to select out people who transmitted *Y. enterocolitia* any better than people who did not. Shortening blood storage interval would have created a major supply problem for blood collectors in the United States and clearly would have had a minimal positive impact on the health of the country. We tolerated the risk of *Y.enterocolitia*.

Graft-versus-host disease has been mentioned in the setting of bone marrow transplants. Graft-versus-host disease also occurs in the setting of blood transfusion. We have long known that it is caused by immunocompetent lymphocytes given to an immunocompromised host, but we now know that it is not just immunocompromised hosts who are at risk. A recipient whose HLA tissue type is similar to that of the blood donor, such as a relative, is also at risk. We now know, especially from studies in Japan, that it may not necessarily be a relative but anyone whose tissue type is similar because of population characteristics. We also know that mortality from transfusion-associated graft-versus-host disease approaches 90 percent. Animal studies show that it takes very few transfused cells to cause this disease. We have known this for years. We could eliminate graft-versus-host disease from blood transfusion essentially by irradiating blood at 2,500 centiGray (cGy). Do we want to do this? No. The costs outweigh the potential benefits. We tolerate this particular risk of blood transfusion for most recipients receiving blood from unrelated donors.

Does allogeneic blood transfusion alter the recipient's immune response? The data go all the way back to the 1960s. We have known for almost 35 years that people who receive blood transfusions develop Fc receptor blocking factors. Their lymphocyte numbers decline, there is a decrease in the helper lymphocytes (CD4), and an increase in the number of the suppressor (CD8) lymphocytes. Those findings were described in hemophiliacs receiving concentrates of protein and clotting factors long before HIV was reported in the blood supply.[72] That clearly muddied the waters a little bit when HIV entered the blood supply.

We also see numbers of activated lymphocytes and down-regulation of antigen-presenting cells. These are all laboratory phenomena, and we have known about them for many years in many populations of transfused individuals. The real question was, do these have any kind of clinical significance? The answer to that is probably yes. We know that there is improved organ allograft survival in transfusion recipients. There is a suggestion that people with cancer who receive allogeneic transfusions have decreased survival or increased recurrence of their malignancy postsurgery. There are data to suggest that people who receive allogeneic blood have increased numbers of postoperative infections. There are also data to suggest that by giving allogeneic transfusions we can

- prevent recurrent abortions that are immune mediated,
- suppress immune inflammatory disease such as ulcerative colitis and Crohn's disease, and
- reactivate latent viruses, such as cytomegalovirus and HIV.

The data go back to the 1970s. The work of Opelz and colleagues[73] on graft survival in patients receiving cadaver kidneys demonstrates that those people who received blood transfusions had better organ graft survival, and there was also a dose response. This suggests that there was an immunosuppressive effect of allogeneic blood. There was great controversy about the data initially, but they have subsequently been confirmed.

Data from 1989, reported in the *New England Journal of Medicine*,[74] showed that if you match the donor and the recipient of allogeneic blood for one haplotype at the DR locus and then look at either kidney or heart transplant recipients, those who received blood transfusion with a match at the DR locus had a better survival of their allograft than did those who received no transfusion or received unmatched blood. This again suggests a fairly potent immunosuppressive effect of blood.

---

[72]Gowperts, E, R deBiasi, R DeVreker (1992). The impact of clotting factor concentrates on the immune system in individuals with hemophilia. *Transfusion Medicine Reviews, 6(1):* 44–53.

[73]Opelz, G, DPS Sengar, MR Mickey, PI Terasaki (1973). Effect of blood transfusion on subsequent kidney transplants. *Transplant Proceedings, 5:* 253–259.

[74]Lagaaji, EL, IPH Hennemann, M Ruigrok, et al. (1989). Effect of one-HLA-DR-antigen-matched and completely HLA-DR-mismatched blood transfusions on suvival of kidney and heart allografts. *New England Journal of Medicine, 321:* 701–705.

At about the same time as these 1989 data, retrospective data were coming in the literature, primarily on colon cancer.[75] In patients who were operated on for colon cancer, those who received allogeneic blood transfusions had a more rapid recurrence of cancer than those who did not. There are about 40 of these studies in the literature, including a series of prospective randomized double-blind studies. At least one of these, appearing in the *American Journal of Clinical Oncology*,[76] suggested that, using autologous blood as a control, those people who received allogeneic blood had more rapid recurrence of cancer and a higher death rate. Several other studies didn't determine that, but there is still a suggestion that this is so. Is that an immunosuppressive effect that we tolerate? I don't know.

There is also the question of postoperative infection. In retrospective reviews of 19 studies, 17 studies found that transfusion was a significant predictor of postoperative infection and in 12 of these 17 studies it was the single best predictor of postoperative infection.[77] Other factors that might be associated with transfusions, such as low hematocrit, blood loss during surgery, duration of surgery, and a host of other factors, when looked at in multivariate analysis, were not significant. Also, those who received autologous blood as a control in matched studies had fewer postoperative infections than those who received allogeneic blood.[78] Is that also an immunosuppressive effect that we tolerate? Five prospective studies of postoperative infection also looked at allogeneic blood transfusion either without controls or with autologous blood as control, or compared allogeneic blood with allogeneic blood that had the white cells taken out of it. In four of these five studies there are fairly strong suggestions that there is an effect of allogeneic transfusion that was associated with more frequent postoperative infections.[79]

Some numbers, but not real data, are available from at patients with AIDS who receive blood transfusions. There was a report from Australia in 1989 suggesting that patients who were at high risk for AIDS had a shorter survival if they received transfusions. That was probably because they were sicker

---

[75] Burrows, L, PI Tarrtar (1982). Effect of blood transfusion on colonic malignancy recurrence rate. *Lancet, ii:* 662.

[76] Heiss, MM, K-W Jauch, CN Delanoff, et al. (1994) Blood transfusion-modulated tumor recurrence: a randomized study of autologous versus homologous blood transfusion in colorectal cancer surgery. *American Journal of Clinical Oncology, 12:* 1859–1863.

[77] Blumberg, N, JM Heal (1988). Transfusion and host defenses against cancer and infection. *Transfusion, 29:* 236.

[78] Heisse, MM, W Mempel, K-W Jauch, et al. (1994). Beneficial effect of autologous blood transfusion on infectious complications after colorectal surgery. *Lancet, 342:* 1328–1333.

[79] Klein, HG (1996). Immunomodulation caused by blood transfusion. In Betz, CD, SN Swisher, S Kleinman, RK Spence, RG Strauss (ed.), *Clinical Practice of Transfusion Medicine.* New York: Churchill Livingstone.

patients. John Ward reported the same kind of phenomenon from the Centers for Diease Control and Pevention (CDC), looking at more rapid progression of AIDS in patients who received blood transfusions.[80] Again, one obvious explanation may be that those who were sicker needed the transfusions.

Additional retrospective studies show decreased survival and increased wasting and bacterial infections in patients with AIDS who received blood transfusion. Michael Busch at Irwin Memorial Blood Center took cells infected with HIV from HIV-positive patients and cocultured these cells with a variety of allogeneic blood cells from healthy blood donors.[81] It is well-known that if you take cells that are infected with a variety of viruses and stimulate them, you can activate the viruses, and the viruses will propagate in the cells. Busch has shown that if you use relatively small amounts of the lectin phytohemagglutinin, you can stimulate these in vivo-infected lymphocytes, and p24 antigen appears in the supernatant of the culture. The next experiment he performed was to take mononuclear cells from healthy donors and coculture them with these HIV-infected lymphocytes. He used different concentrations of mononuclear cells from different healthy donors and found a dose response relationship showing that lymphocytes endogenously infected with HIV were stimulated by coculture with allogeneic mononuclear cells. If you separated out these cells and looked at granulocytes, monocytes, lymphocytes, or unfractionated mononuclear cells, you saw exactly the same kind of phenomenon, but if you took all the white cells out of the allogeneic blood by filtration or washing, or used plasma devoid of lymphocytes, you did not see this phenomenon.

It appears that, in vitro, allogeneic lymphocytes or white cells have some role in the reactivation of latent viruses: cytomegalovirus, HIV, and maybe some oncogenic viruses as well. Lots of leukocytes are included in transfusions of red cells, platelets, and granulocytes. We can remove these if we want to. Is this an important clinical phenomenon, and if so should we attack it with this very large and expensive therapeutic maneuver? Or is this something that we can tolerate until further data are available? The phenomenon of reactivation of latent viruses is now being studied in vivo in a multicenter prospective study sponsored by the National Heart, Lung and Blood Institute. Data are critical when we try to determine which risks are "tolerable," although political decisions often trump data.

---

[80]Ward, JW, MJ Busch, HJ Perkins, et al. (1989). Natural history of transfusion-associated infection with human immunodeficiency virus: Factors influencing the rate of progression of the disease. *New England Journal of Medicine, 321:* 947–951.

[81]Busch, MP, T-H Lee, J Heitman (1992). Allogeneic leukocytes but not therapeutic blood elements induce reactivation of latent HIV-1 infection: Implications for transfusion support of infected patients. *Blood, 80:* 2128–2135.

DISCUSSION

Harold Sox: There is individual decision making, which is trying to decide whether a physician and patient should arrive at a decision to continue the factor concentrate, for instance, or try some alternative approach. There is another type of decision making, which is societal decision making. The individual decision making basically drives the question of whether to treat or not treat, and the societal question drives the question of whether we should clean up the product and get rid of the risk. We need to recognize both of those examples of risk tolerance. When we reach the end of our societal tolerance we begin to devote money to research to get the product cleaned up. Your talk dealt mostly with the question of what risks we do tolerate. At the end you talked about what risks we should tolerate. That last question is probably the one we should be asking.

Elaine Eyster: How does this apply to the situation where there are no suitable alternatives? If the decision is treat or don't treat because there are no suitable alternatives of forms of treatment, then what is one to do?

Harold Sox: Our committee concluded that when there is a great deal of uncertainty, when the stakes are very high, that is the time to completely inform the patient about those risks or lack of knowledge or certainty about the nature of those risks and to engage the patient fully in making a decision that we probably shouldn't try to make for them. That is the strategy that I would recommend.

Elaine Eyster: What if you don't know the extent of the problem though? How do you present that information to the patients so that they can decide?

Harold Sox: We describe the problem as best we can, admit our lack of knowledge such as it is, and bring the patients into the decision. The problem is that we cannot make the decision or solve the problem for them.

Harvey Klein: The question of societal decision making is a very interesting one because society has already decided in terms of HIV infection what it will tolerate in the American blood supply, and that is zero, even though that is not a really rational concept from what we know about the biology of various viruses. It probably isn't a rational concept in terms of cost effectiveness, but society has clearly made that decision. In terms of individual decision making, we now are going to be asking donors about Creutzfeldt-Jakob disease (CJD). Conceivably, we should be informing patients that this is a potential risk in blood transfusion. I would find that very difficult to explain to a patient, because there never has been a case transmitted by transfused blood, but because we are going to be screening our blood supply for CJD, it raises the question of what we do at the patient end.

Elaine Eyster: We are starting to tell our hemophilia patients about CJD. It is one of the most absurd discussions I have ever had, trying to tell them that there might be this problem but we don't know if there is a problem, and although the disease has never been shown to be transmitted in blood, it could be. They need the product, and even the recombinant version might not be totally free of it for all we know.

Lew Barker: I would like to take this a little further into the realm of deep uncertainty. It is becoming evident that we all walk around with a large collection of fragments of retroviral genomes in many of our somatic cells or white cells. These may or may not be dealt with by irradiation or whatever measures we have. They might even be activated, and we obviously transfuse these all the time in people. We have other ways of exchanging lymphocytes, as was learned from infectious mononucleosis some years ago. One of the reasons that I have a problem with "tolerating" the associated but totally unknown risk is that we don't have any idea what to do about it. Other than the attractive alternative of trying to move totally away from allogeneic blood transfusions, I think once we understand jumping genes or whatever they are, there will be something else to concern ourselves with. These may be the problems of the next century associated with allogeneic blood transfusions. Asking people to make these decisions when they cannot really understand these things and we cannot explain them very well is a tough conundrum.

James Allen: Certainly science and literacy are becoming real barriers for us now in terms of communication of risk, communication of what the actual threats are, and what can be done about it. How individuals view risk is very interesting. Risks that they choose, such as riding on a motorcycle with or without a helmet, are risks that individuals freely make for themselves. But when it comes to blood, the media has helped us foster in this country the concept that we should not tolerate any risk in the blood supply. If we move away from allogeneic transfusions, what are we going to substitute them with, and what are the risks associated with that? Whatever it is, maybe we can reduce the risks, but it may take an long time for us to really establish that, given the level of risk that we have at present.

There is also finite risk because we cannot eradicate all risk. In the early 1980s there were two temporally fairly closely linked episodes of bacterial contamination with *Pseudomonas fluorescens* in red cell units coming from the same blood collection center. FDA and CDC got involved in the investigation in that blood center. Subsequently, a third case occurred several months later, and it was from the same source. The investigators went through the whole blood system at that collection center and never could identify a real breach in the process or a potential source of the infection. The problem either went away or never recurred. Whatever that risk is, it is still there. It is an intrinsic risk in the system. We didn't fix anything. We have to acknowledge that there is that baseline level of a potential problem in the system. To the extent that we can identify possible solutions and put in those solutions at a reasonable cost given the resources available, we should do so, but there is always going to be a finite risk of one type or another.

Joseph Fratantoni: Much as science has evolved in the last 20 or 30 years, I think this policy of bringing the patient into the decision has evolved somewhat compared with the early 1980s.

Harold Sox: That is correct. The style of decision making back in the early 1980s was much more weighted toward the physician taking the lead and the patient basically nodding and saying, "Yes, doctor, yes, doctor." For many decisions video disks are now available to inform the patients. When they come to the conference with the physician it is on a reasonably equal footing. Things have changed a lot.

Michael Stoto: The challenge is not only talking honestly about the risk of the uncertainty with a patient but trying to find ways to adapt that in individual circumstances to help the doctor and the patient work together to understand the risks and benefits in a given situation, and what they should do together, given what they know and what they don't know, in order to make a decision about this patient's care. I don't think we are doing it yet, but many are attempting not only to be clear about the uncertainty but really to adapt what is known to individual patients.

V

Risk Communication

A Mental Model Approach to Risk Communication

M. Granger Morgan

When the word risk is mentioned, many of us first think in terms of a single value such as the expected number of deaths or injuries. However, a simple thought experiment can quickly convince us that things are more complicated. Suppose that we are considering introducing a new product. After careful market research we have determined that we can sell a number of them and make a profit, but there will be some net impact, D, on overall US mortality. What sorts of things do we need to know before we decide whether we are justified in introducing this product? In addition to the sign and magnitude of D, most people want to know things such as whether the risk is immediate or delayed, how equally or unequally it is distributed among different people, whether those at risk have any control over their exposure, whether the effects are immediate or delayed, whether there are intergenerational effects, how well the risk is understood, whether it is similar to other risks society already accepts, what the product does, who uses it, and how responsibility and liability will be distributed. As we pursue this simple question we quickly come to understand that risk is a multi-attribute concept. We care about more than just some measure of the number of deaths and injuries.

Slovic, Fischhoff and Lichtenstein[82] have shown that one can group such attributes of risk into three broad factors which allow us to reliably sort risks into a "factor space." People's perceptions of risks, including their beliefs about the need for regulatory intervention, are a strong function of where a risk falls in this space. Risks posed by such common and well known objects and activities as skiing, bicycles, and automobiles appear in the lower left corner

---

[82]Slovic, P, B Fischhoff and S Lichtenstein (1980). Facts and fears: Understanding perceived risk, in Schwing, R and W Albers (ed.), *Societal Risk Assessment*. New York: Plenum.

of the space. In contrast, risks such as those associated with nuclear power, asbestos, and pesticides lie in the upper right hand corner of the space.

Experimental psychologists have discovered that in making judgments, such as the number of deaths from a chance event, people use simple mental rules of thumb called "cognitive heuristics."[83] In many day-to-day circumstances, these serve us very well, but in some instances, they can lead to biases in the judgments we make. This can be a problem for both laypeople and for experts. Three such heuristics are particularly common:

Availability: the probability of an event is judged in proportion to the ease with which people can think of previous occurrences of the event or can imagine such occurrences.

Anchoring and adjustment: the probability judgment is driven by a starting value (anchor) from which people typically do not adjust sufficiently as they consider various relevant factors.

Representiveness: the probability that an object belongs to a particular class is judged in terms of how much it resembles that class.

The design of effective risk communication requires a recognition of the multi-attribute nature of risk, an awareness of the psychology of risk perceptions and judgment under uncertainty, and an analysis of the information needs of the people for whom the communication is intended.

Developing a risk communication has traditionally been a two-step process. First, you find some health or safety specialist who knows a lot about the risk and you ask them what they think people should be told. Then you find someone who is called a "communications expert," who is usually either a writer or someone who works in public relations. You give them the information you got from the health or safety specialist and they decide how they think it should be packaged and delivered.

If you think about it for a while, you will notice that two key things are missing from this traditional approach. First, it doesn't determine systematically what people already know about the risk. People's knowledge is important because they interpret anything you tell them in light of what they already believe. If some of those beliefs happen to be wrong, or misdirected, your message may be misunderstood. It may even lead people to draw conclusions that are exactly the opposite from what you intended. Second, the traditional method doesn't determine systematically the precise information that people need to make the decisions they face. There are formal methods,

---

[83]Kahneman, D, P Slovic and A Tversky (ed.) (1982). *Judgment Under Uncertainty: Heuristics and Biases.* New York: Cambridge University Press. Dawes, RM (1988). *Rational Choice in an Uncertain World.* Orlando, Florida: Harcourt Brace.

decision analysis, that can provide a precise answer to a question such as "what is the minimum set of information I need to make the decisions I care about." Of course, most of us have never heard of decision analysis, and we don't use it in our daily decision making. For various reasons we typically require more than the minimum set of information to make the decisions we face. Yet, when you start reviewing traditional risk communication messages it is amazing how many of them fail to provide even this minimum set of information.

Most of us already have some relevant knowledge and beliefs about any risk that a communication is designed to inform us about. Often we've already heard some specific things about the risk. If we haven't, we've heard about other risks which sound pretty similar. In any event, we have a lot of knowledge about the world around us. We have beliefs about how things work, and about which things are more and less important. When someone tells us about a risk we use all our previous knowledge and beliefs, called our "mental model," in order to interpret what we are being told.

Finding out what someone already knows about a risk means learning about their "mental model." That's easier said than done. We could administer a questionnaire, but people aren't stupid. I have to ask questions about something. As soon as I start putting information in my questions, people are going to start using that information to make inferences and draw conclusions. Pretty soon I'm not going to know if the answers I am getting are telling me about the mental model that the person already had before I started quizzing them, or the new mental model that the person is building because of the all the information I am supplying in my questions.

To overcome these and other problems, we have developed a five-step method for creating, testing and refining risk communication messages:[84]

1. Carefully review scientific knowledge about the risk, and summarize it in terms of a formal diagram called an "influence diagram."
2. Conduct open-ended elicitations of people's beliefs about the hazard, allowing expression of both accurate and inaccurate concepts. Use a "mental model interview protocol" that has been shaped by the influence diagram.
3. Administer structured questionnaires to a larger set of people in order to determine the prevalence of the beliefs encountered in the "mental model" interviews conducted in Step 2.

---

[84]Morgan, MG, B Fischhoff, A Bostrom, L Lave, and C Atman (1992). Communicating risk to the public, *Environmental Science & Technology, 26:* 2048–2056. Bostrom, A, B Fischhoff and MG Morgan (1992). Characterizing mental models of hazardous processes: A methodology and an application to radon, *Journal of Social Issues, 48:* 85–100.

4. Develop a draft risk communication message based on both a decision analytic assessment of what people need to know in order to make informed decisions and a psychological assessment of their current beliefs.

5. Iteratively test and refine successive versions of the risk communication message using open-ended interviews, closed-form questionnaires, and various problem-solving tasks, administered before, during, and after people receive the message.

Suppose that I want to learn about the mental model that someone has for a risk such as the safety of the blood supply. In response to a question like "Tell me about the safety of the blood supply," most people can only talk for a few sentences before they run out of steam. However, those few sentences often contain five or ten different ideas. If the interviewer has been trained to keep track of all the things that are mentioned, they can then go on to ask questions that follow up on each one. For example, they might say "You mentioned that screening blood donors can improve safety. Tell me more about that. . ." By systematically following up on all the concepts that the subject introduces, a well-trained interviewer can often sustain a conversation about the risk for 10 to 20 minutes, introducing no new ideas of their own. Only in a later stage of the interview will the interviewer go on to ask questions about other key ideas which the subject did not bring up on their own.

By conducting a number of interviews of this sort, we can begin to build up some sense of what people know and believe about a risk. Then in step three of the process, using a closed-form questionnaire, we can determine the relative frequency with which various beliefs actually occur in the general public.

Every time that we have conducted mental model interview studies to prepare a risk communication, we have learned surprising and important things which have had a major effect on the message we developed. Among the most important insights have come from some of the common misconceptions. For example, in studies of radon, we learned that a significant number of Americans believe that once they get radon in their house, the house becomes permanently contaminated and there is nothing they can do about it. Of course, this is not true. Radon is a radioactive gas that decays into various particles which become nonradioactive in a matter of hours. Thus, if the source of radon gas can be closed off, all of the resulting radioactivity will soon be gone from the home. This is an important part of any risk communication message, because if you test your home for radon and find elevated concentrations, you can take various steps to prevent the radon from entering the home and thus reduce or eliminate the risk. How could people think that a house that has radon is permanently contaminated? Probably they are extrapolating from other things they know. They have heard about radioactive waste from power plants and bomb factories that remains dangerous for 100,000 years. They also may have heard of houses that have become chemically contaminated when they were sprayed by very long lasting pesticides. They make a reasonable extrapolation (which in this case happens to be wrong) that radon is like these other cases. This is the sort of misconception that it is critical to know about if you are going to design an effective risk communication. When EPA designed their first *Citizen's Guide to Radon*, which was mailed to citizens all over the country, they didn't know about this common misconception. Their central message was "You should test your house for radon." However, many people who believe that radon permanently contaminates a house would probably be inclined to ignore this message, figuring they are better off not knowing whether their house has a high concentration of radon. For example, if they don't know, they could sell their house some time in the future with a clear conscience.

In summary, in order to develop an effective risk communication one must recognize that risk is a multi-attribute concept. Building on the literature on risk perception and judgment under uncertainty, one should learn what people already know about the risk at hand, first through open-ended mental model interviews, and then through closed-form questionnaires. On the basis of this, and a careful assessment of the information people need to make on the decisions they face, a first draft of the communication can be developed. However, there is no such thing as an expert in risk communication. The only way to be certain that a message works, that it is understood in the way that it is intended, is to try it out on real people. By using a variety of methods, including one-on-one read aloud protocols and focus groups, the message can be iteratively refined. Test it; refine it; test it again. Don't stop until it works.

DISCUSSION

Henrik Bendixen: How do you know when risk communication works effectively?

M. Granger Morgan: One strategy is to present people with a hypothetical situation and ask them what actions they would take. For example, we did a three-way study with the first version of the EPA *Citizen's Guide to Radon* and two brochures we developed from the results of our work. In terms of simple recall, regurgitating the facts, the three did roughly comparably. Then we asked participants to respond to a question such as: "You have a neighbor who has just measured radon levels in their home of 10 picocuries per liter. What advice do you give them?" The people who read either of the brochures we developed were able to give direct, cogent, and correct advice, but the people who had read only the EPA brochure had a lot of trouble. They basically were not able to provide an answer.

Risk Communication: Building Credibility

Caron Chess

The following true story illustrates the difficulty of relying only on numbers to explain risk. A high-ranking government official was speaking to a public meeting of hundreds of people about a proposal for a hazardous waste incinerator in their neighborhood. The audience was told that the incinerator would pose only a 1 in 1 million risk of an increased death from cancer. The crowd's response: "We hope you are the one."[85]

If this agency representative had been able to explain more eloquently the 1 in a million risk, would people have said, "Oh, now we understand. We will graciously accept your incinerator." The answer, of course, is no. Nonetheless, senior scientists, administrators, and public health officials seek to improve their explanations of the risk numbers in hopes that the public will yield to experts' judgments. These experts are overemphasizing the impact of explanations of the mortality and morbidity data. I suggest that this and other environmental communication issues apply to communication about blood safety. In the following few pages I discuss three myths that scientists and policy makers believe about explaining risk and propose alternative approaches.

ROLE OF INFORMATION

One myth is that information changes behavior, while in reality, information has little association with behavior. Although scientific experts are very careful to limit extrapolation beyond the data when dealing with their own disciplines, they tend go beyond the social science data (and sometimes go where no social scientist has gone before).

---

[85] Hance, BJ, C Chess, PM Sandman (1988). *Improving Dialogue with Communities: A Risk Communication Manual for Government.* Trenton: New Jersey Department of Environmental Protection.

Experts who are not social scientists have in mind a model about the role of information that is flawed. Many non-social scientists erroneously believe that if you give people information about risk, they will change their attitudes and then they will change their behaviors. However, empirical research suggests that increased knowledge about technology is not necessarily associated with support of that technology. For example, in a review of research on perception of the risks of nuclear energy, about one-half of the studies show that supporters of nuclear power know more factual knowledge than opponents. The other studies show that opponents of nuclear power know more information than supporters or that opponents and supporters have equal amounts of information.[86]

In the health education field there is an evolving consensus that knowledge has a weak link to behavior. For example, high school kids right now can pass tests of their AIDS knowledge, but they have not changed their behavior dramatically. Likewise, women may know that they are at risk for AIDS if they have unprotected sex with a partner who is HIV infected. That knowledge does not mean that women will insist that their partners use condoms.

Advertisers who want to change behavior talk about messages and appeals rather than information: appeals to status, social approval, sex appeal and so forth. Similarly, those who attempt to change behavior for the social good, dubbed *social marketing*, develop communication strategies and messages based on what motivates people to change their behavior.[87] For instance, years ago antismoking campaigns were replete with images of anatomically explicit photographs of damage to lungs caused by smoking. Somewhat later, there was a complete change in message, based on research about what motivates teenagers' behavior: television ads featured Brooke Shields telling kids that it was uncool to smoke.

When those of you in the blood industry are considering how to increase the pool of donors, you need to think in terms of social marketing. For example, the message that donating blood cannot lead to HIV infection, while a seemingly logical response to public fears, needs to be supported by empirical research on questions such as: To what extent does fear of HIV affect those people who have a record of donating blood? Does that fear largely affect those whose psychological portrait suggests that they would be donors? Or does it largely affect those who would be unlikely to give blood under any conditions? If the fear does affect people otherwise likely to give

---

[86] Johnson, BB (1993). Advancing understanding of knowledge's role in lay risk perception. *Risk: Issues in Health, Safety, and the Environment, 4:* 189–212.

[87] For example, Rice, RE, CK Atkin (1989). *Public Communication Campaigns.* Newbury Park: Sage.

blood, how well is their fear reduced by the message about the lack of connection between HIV and blood donation?

Some existing empirical research begins to answer this question by distinguishing the attitudes of those who donate blood from those who do not donate blood.[88] According to one study, people who give blood tend to associate blood donation with generosity, civic mindedness, and usefulness as well as feelings of assurance and relaxation.

Those who do not donate blood connect donation with illness and discomfort. This study suggests that motivating donors might build on their positive associations, not merely factual information about the lack of connection between giving blood and AIDS. Attracting more donors requires more such research to determine feelings about blood donation, to develop potential messages based on that research, and to test those messages.

If you want to change behavior, for example, encouraging people to donate blood or to become repeat donors, you need to understand their motivations, biases, and beliefs. This same need for understanding is also essential to discouraging people who continue to donate blood, even though they know they are HIV-positive or that they may be at risk of HIV infection. If you are going to communicate with those individuals, you want to know what their attitudes and beliefs are and what motivates them to behave in this manner.

When you do provide information, you should consider what your audience wants to know, not merely what you want to tell them. To provide this information, you need to know what your audience thinks is important—and knowing your audience requires further research.

THE ROLE OF RISK NUMBERS

Scientific experts tend to subscribe to a second myth: the public is influenced largely by the risk numbers. However, as the previous discussion suggests, individuals are influenced by factors other than the risk data. A true story about a prominent Environmental Protection Agency risk assessor illustrates the influence of other variables.[89] The risk assessor was in the hospital for tests, including one that had a slight risk of causing kidney failure. He found that more sophisticated diagnostic equipment, without the potential risk, existed at a hospital across town. He decided to take an ambulance to the other hospital to use the more sophisticated diagnostic equipment—even

---

[88]Beckler, SJ (1989). Scales for the measurement of attitudes towards blood donation. *Transfusion, 29:* 401–404.

[89]Siegel, B (1987). Managing risks: Sense and science. *Los Angeles Times*, July 5, I 28.

though his wife pointed out to him that the risk of the ambulance trip across town was greater than the risk of kidney failure. The risk assessor chose a familiar risk (a ride across town) rather than the less familiar one (the unfamiliar, potentially harmful technology). The risk assessor acknowledged that he did not make his personal decision by the numbers, even though he knew it was illogical.

Now how does this story relate to the field of blood donation? People tend to be less fearful of the familiar risks than the unfamiliar risks, regardless of the risk numbers.[90] According to the literature on risk perception, there are also psychological rules of thumb that influence perceptions more than the risk numbers. One rule of thumb, "the availability heuristic," suggests that the most vivid images on our psychic landscape influence how we see risk.[91] Therefore, because homicides get a great deal of publicity, most of us see homicides as a more frequent cause of death than it is. Similarly, people are less influenced by numbers such as a 1 in 400,000 risk of contracting HIV from a blood transfusion, than they are by the powerful images of famous AIDS victims such as Elizabeth Glaser or Ryan White.

THE ROLE OF RISK COMPARISONS

Risk comparisons reflect the tremendous desire on the part of scientists to compare risks that are not part of daily lives (such as the risk of contracting HIV from blood donation) with familiar risks that people take every day. Often, the goal is to suggest that everyday risks, such as driving, are more risky than those risks that people fear, such as donating or receiving blood. However, despite the interest in using risk comparisons, few studies have explored the impacts of such comparisons. The results of one suggested that the risk comparison did not have any effect when subjected to emotional criticism of the comparison.[92]

Another study asked subjects to vote on their willingness to accept a hazardous waste incinerator.[93] The risk of the facility was compared to smoking a dozen cigarettes. When the comparison was used, more people said they would oppose the incinerator than when the comparison was not used.

---

[90] For example, Slovic, P (1987). Perception of risk. *Science 236:* 280–285.

[91] Kahneman, D, P Slovic, A Tversky (ed.) (1982). *Judgment under Uncertainty: Heuristics and Biases.* New York: Cambridge University Press.

[92] Slovic, P, N Krause, V Covello (1990). What should we know about making risk comparisons? *Risk Analysis, 10:* 389–392.

[93] Freudenberg, W, J Rursch (1994). The risk of putting numbers in context: A cautionary tale. *Risk Analysis 14:* 949–958.

The research did not suggest why the risk comparison had this impact. However, the lesson is that if you want to use a risk comparison, you better conduct research on its influence.

SOURCES OF CONFLICT

Yet another myth subscribed to by scientific experts is that conflict is due to the public's lack of understanding of a subject, while in reality, trust and values often play much larger roles. One model for societal decision making values information as the most critical element, while another values the importance of participatory decision making. The premise of the first model is that cost/benefit analysis and risk trade-offs are acceptable ways to make societal decisions. This model assumes that decisions should be made on a scientific basis and that science is objective. The second model suggests that decisions should be premised on the basis of equity and fairness rather than merely risk.[94] These are obviously two very different equations for decision making. Is one right and the other wrong? I would submit you that the difference in the models is a question of values, not rightness or wrongness.

The second model of decision making explains how conflict about scientific issues may have roots in the lack of trust in those who have decision-making authority. According to one review of the literature, trust is asymmetrical.[95] It is easy for experts to lose trust; it is far harder to gain it. Once trust is broken, it is difficult to recover. Also, sources of bad news are more credible than sources of good news, at least in our culture, and bad news carries more weight than good news.

These findings from the literature were applied to a study in which participants were asked to respond to statements concerning activities of a hypothetical local nuclear power plant.[96] The one condition that was found to increase trust significantly referred to a local board with the power to shut down the nuclear power plant if it did not function as promised. This finding underlines the importance of control to individuals confronted with situations they view as risky. Similarly, a literature review concerning siting of hazardous waste facilities, which was conducted for the trade association for

---

[94]For example, Vaughan, E. (1995). The significance of socioeconomic and ethnic diversity for the risk communication process. *Risk Analysis, 15:* 169–180.

[95]Slovic, P (1993). Risk, trust and democracy. *Risk Analysis 13:* 675–681.

[96]*Ibid.*

the nuclear power industry, concluded that public participation seemed to increase the likelihood of acceptance of siting.[97]

What are the implications of such research for the blood industry? One, you need to focus on increasing trust, not merely conveying data. Two, you need to discuss more about the process of how decisions are made and who makes them. And three, you need to consider involving those who are affected by the decisions in the decision-making process.

Extrapolation from the environment data can make this link more explicit: if I were a hemophiliac I might be less interested in hearing from you the current risk data than knowing what you are doing to reduce my risk, to protect me from whatever risk is out there. I am not going to merely weigh the benefit of my getting plasma versus the risk of not getting it. I am also likely to consider: To what extent did the blood industry protect my life? Did they do as much as they could have?

If you want to build trust, one of your hopes may be involving other credible sources in the decision making. If you think you need trust in order to make these policy decisions, you may have a hard time if you make decisions solely on the basis of risk data without consideration of the elements that may affect trust.

Paul Slovic's research[98] suggests that credibility is made up of two components: competence and trust. Do you know how to do what you do? Can you be trusted? I submit to the blood industry that you may need to change perceptions of your competence and your trustworthiness and that information alone will not change those perceptions.

DISCUSSION

Question from the audience: So are you saying we need someone like Brooke Shields as a spokesperson?

Caron Chess: I do not know enough about perceptions of the blood supply to know what image is going to change people's behavior toward donating blood or the blood industry. But I would also consider how you are framing the problem. I would look not only at how to increase the donor pool but also whether to educate doctors to reduce the number of transfusions (since the Institute of Medicine briefing book suggested that doctors may overuse transfusions). I also might look at people who are repeat donors and try to

---

[97]Richards, M. (1993). Siting industrial facilities: Lessons from the social science literature. International Conference for the Advancement of Socioeconomics, March 26–28, 1993, New York.

[98]Slovic, P (1993), *op cit.*

find out what type of person gives blood routinely. It might be easier to increase the number of repeat donors than to increase the donor pool. That is, I try to look at the range of questions before I frame the research or the campaign.

Question from the audience: What you are saying is that we can increase donation by appropriate techniques?

Caron Chess: Yes, but, and this is a major but, I think social marketing campaigns can only be done effectively when there is societal consensus. We can conduct social marketing campaigns about smoking cessation and using seat belts; we can market routine mammograms and blood donation. But you cannot conduct social marketing, I think, ethically or in a way that would increase trust, to fight more regulation or more testing of the blood supply. Of course, as an industry you can battle those issues in other ways—which might further erode your credibility. You can, however, deal with the availability of blood as a social marketing issue.

Question from the audience: I think there are cases where risk-taking behavior changes after the fact. I am trying to figure out why that happens. Eating habits, for example, might be an example. Has that happened or is social marketing always there as the driving force to positive change?

Caron Chess: In order to conduct smoking cessation campaigns I suspect that researchers had to talk to some kids who stopped smoking to try to figure out why they did, although social marketing alone is not sufficient to explain all behavioral changes.

M. Granger Morgan: I would argue for a slightly larger role for information than you have. I do not disagree at all in terms of immediate action, but I would argue that in the context of something such as smoking, there has been a long, gradual diffusion effect, and in the absence of the information the diffusion effect probably would not have occurred. We probably would not have seen the social transformation we saw. I doubt anybody can describe the actual causal mechanisms that gave rise about 8 or 10 years ago to the social tipping that suddenly resulted in the decision that the time has come to do something about smoking. Many of us are hoping that we are seeing the early signs of a similar social tipping with respect to handguns in this society.

Caron Chess: I agree. Certainly there is a diffusion effect with information. Information also has an agenda-setting effect. What I am suggesting is that people who are scientists sometimes overrely on conveying information to transform people's consciousness and behavior. I am not saying throw the information out the window.

Question from the audience: You said that once trust is lost it is nearly impossible to regain. I think the public has largely lost trust in the American blood supply system, for whatever reason. Are there strategies that have been used to regain trust? Is there a stepwise process that over time one can engage in to regain trust, given that you said it is nearly impossible?

Caron Chess: Human beings are difficult, because we don't respond like rats. Something like trust is fairly complex. In the environmental field the question of regaining trust is also a very live one because our environmental institutions have lost credibility. The question is: How do institutions regain credibility? One of the elements that is being looked at is stakeholder involvement. If there is not trust in the decision makers, maybe you need to involve the skeptics. Different approaches to participation are being tried around the country.

Question from the audience: Do you know of any example that has been studied where trust was lost and then regained? Does Tylenol count?

Caron Chess: If Tylenol had come out and said, "It is not us; we are the good guys; there is nothing to worry about," they might have faced an erosion of trust and then needed to increase their credibility. Instead, right from the beginning their chief executive officer, and this is a classic case that is used in the literature time and time again, said, "I do not care about the statistics. I do not care what you lawyers say. We are going to be more proactive." So Tylenol lost some of its market share but then regained it. I think that loss in market share was due more to people's fear of being victims of random poisoning than loss of trust in the people who make Tylenol.

Question from the audience: Ford recovered from Pinto and they did it by behaving in a trustworthy way for a long, long time and also pounding away on safety messages.

Henrik Bendixen: A more modern example is Intel. They may be having some trouble.

Caron Chess: Yes, and that shows the more cynical approach taken by companies such as Exxon and Union Carbide—the "It's not my fault approach" that goes something like, "What? Me? Us? No, you are mistaken." Then comes the backpedaling and saying, "Okay, well, maybe we do have some responsibility." Both companies lost a tremendous amount of credibility. The so-called issue-attention cycle[99] is also involved in retrieving credibility. I think if people do not focus on an issue for a long enough period of time, the involved company is not on people's mind, and over time the memory of the company's action fades. Finally, acting in ways people perceive as trustworthy may be at least as important as talking about safety.

However, you people in the blood industry really blew it. The infected populations are not going to forget too soon. I think that what you need to do is to listen to your detractors' messages. In environmental situations where win-win solutions are being sought, issues have been going to mediation. I am not suggesting that the blood industry should necessarily go to mediation. What I am suggesting is that perhaps you need to look at alternative approaches to problem solving and alternative ways of dealing with your detractors. What I would not be doing if I were in the blood industry is beating up on the Food and Drug Administration. Why? Because people are going to feel more safe if they feel that there is a good watchdog out there. Also, if I were in your shoes I would be funding researchers to find out how people perceive blood donation and the blood industry.

Richard K. Spence: Is it possible to overcome some of the problem of trust by making the risk more acceptable to people? If you point out the benefits to transfusion, how do people buy into it? We know it is risky to drive a car, less so than to fly an airplane, but perhaps people drive because the benefit is better.

Caron Chess: The benefits to whom and under whose value system? There are situations in which all the money imaginable, according to empirical research, would not get people to accept a hazardous waste facility because money was not as important to them as control of their lives. There were other issues at stake other than more traditional weighing of costs and benefits. While I understand your point about the benefits of transfusion, if I were a hemophiliac I am not sure that your statistics about benefits would give me comfort. What I would want to know is: "What are you doing to make me safe these days. What kinds of decisions are you making and on what basis?"

---

[99]Downs, A (1972). Up and down with ecology: The issue-attention cycle. *The Public Interest, 28:* 38–50.

Attitudes Toward Risk: The Right to Know and the Right to Give Informed Consent

Jonathan D. Moreno

I am a philosopher by training. Because I work in medical ethics at a medical center, I often think about issues of trust. To a very great extent my field is directly a result of the gradual erosion of trust in the medical profession that has occurred in the American community at large. The buzz word that is used in bioethics is paternalism, to refer to doctors who think that they know better than patients do what is good for the patients. The peculiar consequence has been that another expert group has been created, namely, the bioethicists, who so far have not been burned by any horrible scandals that have undermined the public confidence in what bioethicists have to say.

The social scientist is often supposed to give a prescription that would solve the problem. Bioethicists are also expected to give such a prescription in a way that a natural scientist would not be expected to do. When that happens I think of my mother-in-law's advice to me just before I was married. She said to me, "Look, I am not going to tell you what to do, I am just going to tell you the right thing to do." I try not to tell my colleagues what to do.

I want to share with you a couple of thoughts about something I am doing this year that has made me think about risk in a new way. This year I am working for the President's Advisory Committee on Human Radiation Experiments, a group of 13 experts and 1 nonexpert, to give it legitimacy, in the fields of nuclear medicine, radiation oncology, ethics, history, and law. There has been a great deal of public attention to 50 years of human radiation experiments, as they are somewhat awkwardly called, paid for with federal funds.

A lot of people in medicine use radioisotopes, and they are very unhappy about all the attention. Many feel that people will have a misunderstanding about the actual risks of radiation compared to all the other risks to which we are exposed. I have had people in nuclear medicine complain to me that because radioisotopes are relatively very safe, especially when used in tracer doses, and that it is really people who use external radiation, X-rays, who ought to be studied more carefully.

Along these lines, besides such straightforward clinical uses of radiation, the Advisory Committee is also studying the fact that federal nuclear sites like the one in Hanford, Washington, and possibly others, had engaged over the years in what are called intentional releases of ionizing radiation, radioactive iodine and other substances, into the atmosphere. This has caused a great deal of concern in places such as Seattle whose population might have have received some of this extra radiation in the atmosphere.

It turns out that an intentional release called the Green Run probably contributed only 1 percent of the radiation that was added to the atmosphere from Hanford in that year. Yet, what is important to people is not necessarily that 1 percent but the reason for that 1 percent. Many believe that the reason had something to do with secret government activity, with knowing how to measure radiation when we were worried about radiation warfare, or maybe the way that radiation would be taken into the plant life and get into the food chain. It is not so much the numbers in many cases that matter to people as it is the background story, the reason that people were exposed to risk, how things happened the way they did, and the decision process that people went through. The fact that it was done in secret simply makes people more anxious and thus affects the way that people assess the nature of these specific risks.

I will very briefly say some things about what people in medical ethics have to say about risk issues and the so-called right to know. I feel very insecure when I give talks before people in the blood services because in bioethics we have done a fair job of dealing with issues in the clinical setting and in research ethics. Theoretically, we are pretty good at dealing with those kinds of issues analytically.

However, when you get into public health ethics we are not doing as well. We have a very limited framework of analysis. The blood area is one that is very difficult for us to cope with because the risks and benefits associated with transfusion or with retrospective studies such as look-backs are so hard to know. In many cases, harms as well as benefits are remote and the bioethical conceptual framework is not well designed for those kinds of problems. We are struggling with the same kinds of uncertainty problems that you are struggling with with respect to blood.

That we in bioethics are limited in our ability to help you does not mean that I will not tell you what I think you ought to do. The conceptual framework that people in bioethics have developed might be called an autonomy-based framework. It is founded on the idea of personal self-determination. The principles that you hear from bioethicists are often called our mantra: autonomy, beneficence, nonmaleficence, and justice. Autonomy comes first. The ethical framework that we have derived from the clinical and research setting is an autonomy-based framework. It is very difficult to know theoretically how to trump self-determination. That is very important from your point of view, because if autonomy, also called self-determination, is more important than any other ethical consideration then clearly people have a right to know just about anything and everything that could possibly go into their decision making so that they can continue to preserve and promote their own self-determination.

This kind of framework seems to work fairly well in the clinical setting. It probably works even better in research, especially when you are talking about research that will not benefit the subjects, normal healthy volunteers, for example. However, in the public health area autonomy can generate terrible problems unless you are at the extreme case of a highly contagious disease in which it is quite clear that the benefit to the wider community ought to trump personal autonomy.

In New York we recently had the example of HIV-related multiple-drug-resistant tuberculosis (TB). This was an easy one to resolve because most of these people were prisoners. There was not a lot of argument about the need to isolate them. There was not even a lot of argument about invading their privacy and doing direct observation of therapy to make sure that they actually took this unpleasant medication to be certain that we do not develop new strains of drug-resistant TB.

When you get to an area such as AIDS, for example, a disease that has to do with intimate behaviors that are infectious but not contagious, you are dealing with a condition that strains what classical liberalism understands is the boundary between the private and the public. Is decision making with respect to the control of HIV a private matter or a public matter? Diseases that are infectious but not highly contagious tend to straddle the public-private boundary. We do not really know very well how to deal with those kinds of issues.

An example of the way that bioethics tried to deal with this public-private boundary problem and the dominance of autonomy in its typical analytic framework in the AIDS era concerned a problem that came up about 10 years ago. What would you do if you had a coded list of blood donors and you knew which donors had given you HIV-positive units? You had collected that list for contact tracing or to develop a sense of the epidemiology of the disease. Once you have such a list, do you have to go to the donors and inform them that they are HIV positive? I am sure you remember these days very well. The autonomy-based conclusion was that if you have such a list, if as the person in authority you know the name of someone who has given such a unit, then you have an obligation to respect the autonomy of that person and share the information with that person.

However, what if you had never organized such a list and you are only considering making such a list? Do you have an obligation to make a list, to identify the units that are infected so that you can tell these donors that they were infected? The answer given to that was no. You may have an obligation for public health reasons to find out who gave the HIV-positive units, but you do not have a moral obligation. Why not? Because there is nothing you can necessarily do for that person therapeutically once you tell him or her. The counterargument was that maybe you could at least prevent that person from infecting somebody else. That goes back to a public health obligation. We got to this very peculiar point in an autonomy-based analysis in which once you had the list of identified HIV-positive donors then you had to go tell them. But if you had not made such a list in the first place, then autonomy did not obligate you to go out and make that list. To many people this kind of analysis is and continues to be unsatisfactory, but it was the conclusion that was generally reached in the bioethics community at the time that these lists were being assembled.

Let me walk you through the way that an analysis of right-to-know issues is supposed to take place in contemporary bioethics. I want to precede this walkthrough by just pointing out that the data on the desire among cancer patients to know their diagnosis indicate that the desire is very high. Basically, 90 percent of cancer patients say that they want to know their diagnosis, especially if it is a grave diagnosis.[100]

A day or two after they are told the information relative to their diagnosis, half of cancer patients retain one or two relevant facts from the clinical interview in which the nature of their disease was explained to them. There is a significant gap between how much people want to know and feel that they have a right to know and how much they can actually retain.

Nonetheless, the vast majority of patients in this culture say that they want to know virtually everything that is relevant to their disease. So with that background, how would we understand the right to know in bioethics? The answer is that people have a right to run the course of their own lives and they need information in order to do that. That does not mean that you have the obligation to go out and get the information. It does mean that if you have it, you have to share it with them because it is something they need to know. It will change the way that they think about their future and change their decision making.

The problem with this idea of autonomy is that it comes from multiple sources. When you get to finely tuned problems, such as whether we should continue syphilis testing as a surrogate for lifestyles, this multiply sourced

---

[100] Alfidi, RJ (1971). Informed consent: a study of patient reaction. *Journal of the American Medical Association, 216:* 1325.

notion of autonomy is not necessarily all that helpful. One source for the idea of autonomy is legal cases. There have been a string of legal cases mostly having to do with surgery from the early 1900s to the 1960s, in which surgeons removed tissues without telling people they were going to do that or why they were going to do that. Gradually, the doctrine of informed consent came along through the courts. Strangely, but importantly, the notion that people have a right to be informed before surgery is not necessarily followed by the notion that failure to inform is something that has to be paid for by the surgeon or his or her insurance company. In other words, it is clear that, in theory at least, patients are supposed to be informed before surgical procedures. It is not at all clear that a patient who is not informed can collect damages unless he or she suffers some injury at the same time in that procedure.

We also get the notion of autonomy, of course, from various philosophers, especially from Immanuel Kant. What Kant thought autonomy is is different from what most of us think it is. Kant thought that autonomy meant following the moral law. Not too many Americans think that autonomy means following the moral law; rather, they think that it means following their preferences. That is not what the philosophical tradition thinks of autonomy.

We also get notions concerning autonomy from the many political and sociological changes we have gone through, from the gradual transformation of patients into consumers. We also get it, of course, from research ethics scandals: Tuskegee, Willowbrook, and the Brooklyn Jewish Chronic Disease Hospital are among the most famous of these.[101]

Let me apply some of the elements of this multiply sourced notion of autonomy to the notion of risk. The term *risk* is to a very great extent a placeholder for the likelihood of something bad happening or the likelihood of something bad happening to *me*, which is even worse. The idea of risk is also ambiguous, not differentiating between the likelihood of a harm and the severity of that harm. In fact, many people who write about risk-benefit these days prefer to talk about harm-benefit.

Our thin theory of autonomy that is multiply-sourced does reasonably well with risks that are likely, severe, and known to others, such as getting an HIV-positive unit of blood, especially when the potential offsetting benefits of not being informed are remote or ambiguous. Thus, in the clinical setting cancer patients must be informed that a bone marrow transplant is unlikely to succeed (although they often do not appreciate that), will cause discomfort, and may itself lead to death. In the research setting one must inform subjects that an innovative treatment will probably not help them (although they very often

---

[101]Faden, R, T Beauchamp (1986). *A History and Theory of Informed Consent.* New York: Oxford.

appreciate that that is true), but that what will be learned may help somebody else.

How then does an autonomy-based bioethics that is multiply-sourced and pretty thin assess the very refined specific questions that come up in the field of blood services? How does a thin theory of autonomy help people to assess informing people about harms that are remote, albeit severe, and perhaps known to others? Recall one of the other principles in the bioethics mantra, which is beneficence. Imagine that we have a case in which the benefits of informing will be very great for a few, though minor when spread out over the aggregate of the community, and justice will perhaps suffer—the third principle in the mantra—because health care resources will now have been distributed. They will have been spent on great benefits for a very few but have relatively no effect on the vast majority of people.

Even if you had this kind of situation in which the benefits are great for a few and justice is perhaps violated because only a few people enjoy these very expensive benefits—the money could be better spent elsewhere—in an autonomy-based bioethic that is not necessarily conclusive. An autonomy-based bioethical theory may obligate people to spend a lot of money on a very few and therefore benefit them but leave the vast majority untouched, and risk the problem of maldistribution of precious social resources.

That is pretty much where we are. Our bioethical theory is no better than the general public's attitude. When the general public reads about or learns about an exemplary individual case, there is a reflex to rescue, and that reflex to rescue the known victim does not have a clear answer in what bioethical theory has to offer in these kinds of problematic situations.

A number of different criteria have been used in the clinical setting to determine the limits of the right to know. Doctors want to know how meager a risk they to talk to their patients about? How much do they have to tell them, and so forth? Informing about every possible risk looks crazy beyond a certain point.

A number of other standards have been used, because autonomy-based bioethics leads to this potentially crazy result in which even the most remote risks have to be disclosed. One is the reasonable person standard, that is, what a reasonable person would want to know. However, we know, of course, that risk assessment is not reasonable and is mostly apprehended through famous, exemplary cases.

The second standard is what would this particular person want to know. This is popular in bioethics because it conforms to an autonomy-based theory, in that you respect the autonomy of this particular patient. That might work if you have a long-term doctor-patient relationship and so know the values of your patient, but it is unlikely to work in the health maintenance organization (HMO) setting. In public health it does not have any usefulness at all.

The third possibility is whatever the experts think plus the precedent of what they decided to do before. That has some value legally. Arguably it has moral importance because it suggests a policy is consistent from one case to another. That is important. Similar cases are being treated similarly. Unfortunately, it might also beg the question and perpetuate unreasonable previous policies and standards.

Suppose we accept the last standard: what the experts think, plus what they decided before. That criterion may be modified by a special fact that makes blood services so interesting and unique. That is, in your field trust is perhaps uniquely important. You know pretty fast if you have lost the public trust because people stop showing up to donate or because the various interest groups that are recipients of blood give you feedback pretty fast.

It is the case that expert judgment plus precedent plus bending over backwards prudently, if not morally, to overinform about risks is the best formula that we can come up with with respect to the issues that concern you. I want to leave a place for expert judgment. I want to encourage you to sustain a level of consistency about the way that you approach each case, and, to bend over backwards, if needed, to "hyperinform" because in the last instance the issues of blood are more sensitive to problems of trust than are other issues in health care.

I do have one thing to add to the issues of expert judgment, precedent and hyperinforming. There are some indications that financial issues are affecting health policy recommendations in a way that they have not explicitly affected them before. As an example, a few months ago the National Cancer Institute (NCI) changed its policy on recommendations concerning routine annual breast cancer screening, increasing the age from 40 to 45 to 50. Some people have argued in the literature that this decision was transparently a cost-containment policy initiative. They note that when Samuel Broder, the Dierector of the NCI, testified on this before Congress, he seemed to be uncomfortable. During questioning he said that was a policy that he recommended in his position at the NCI. When he was asked what he would recommend to a 40-year-old patient who perhaps had a family history of breast cncer, he said he would tell her to get screened.

This whole discussion may be different 5 years from now. When we are talking especially about doing look-backs, cost issues may be much more salient than they ever have been before in this kind of analysis.

In summing up, I would say, first, that in blood services, warnings of prospective risks to recipients of blood should probably favor what many would regard as overinforming, because of society's autonomy orientation and expectations, prudence, and the fact that trust is such a delicate quality.

Second, studies of retrospective risks are only morally obligatory when the problem is serious and an effective therapy is available. When such studies are undertaken and specific at-risk individuals are identified, then those individuals have to be informed.

Finally, I suggest to you that decisions to undertake look-backs will undoubtedly be more affected by cost considerations in the future than they have been in the past.

DISCUSSION

Henrik Bendixen: I would offer one comment. Several years ago Joshua Lederburg chaired a committee[102] which predicted that there would be more new diseases coming along. As we speak about trust and communicating risk, the most important thing that we could do in the next few years is to look to the future, to think about what the situation might be 5 or 10 years from now and to mobilize in the best possible way to be ready for the next one when it comes, because come it will.

M. Granger Morgan: Suppose, in fact, a medical facility and a blood system in some region starts providing elaborate information about risk, while another facility and system does not provide that elaborate information. Suppose I then run a parallel study and discover that for a set of standard procedures the mortality risk is significantly higher in the informed population because many people are foregoing the use of blood. Do you want to tell me about that from the point of view of a medical bioethicist?

Jonathan Moreno: This is very much the same kind of question that clinicians have raised over the years when people have argued that they ought to tell people about the downside of chemotherapy, for example. Not only is it potentially inhumane to do that when there are very few alternatives, but you might scare them away and create more disease and a worse outcome. I do not know if the experience that we have had in the clinical setting can be applied to the kind of aggregate communities that we are talking about in blood. However, in the clinical setting patients feel that they know the potential harms of what the physician is recommending and have decided to accept the physician's recommendation. It is a good research question. Maybe we could do a controlled study at two centers and try it out.

Thomas Zuck: There may be a way that we can get at it with the Gann Act in California, which requires a very detailed formulation of what you have to

---

[102]Institute of Medicine (1992). (ed.) (1992). *Emerging Infections: Microbial Threats to Health in the United States.* Washington, D.C.: National Academy Press.

tell patients and what the alternatives are. Three or four states now have Gann Acts. Could we somehow compare outcomes in those places that have Gann Acts for specific kinds of procedures with outcomes in states that do not?

Kenrad Nelson: I would like to raise a question related to blood bank practices that tails on the previous question. Autologous donations now have been promoted by physicians and the general public. This may be an important way to reduce the risks of transfusion. But also there has been some movement to increase the use of directed donation. That is, you have a relative or somebody who specifically donates for you or for a given person. Some studies suggest that the prevalence of markers of hepatitis, HIV, and other infectious agents is significantly higher among the directed donors than it is among the general pool of donors. It relates to the fact that if you have pressure from a relative to donate a unit of blood for the family you may be less inclined to admit a behavioral risk for HIV. Therefore, the risk from a directed donation is higher. I was recently visited by a lawyer who was representing a patient who developed hepatitis C after a transfusion and now had chronic hepatitis and cirrhosis. His legal argument was going to be that the person was not told by the blood bank or by the surgeon about the possibility of a directed donation. If he had known, he could have made the decision to ask a relative to donate and this would have been safer. I said, yes, he could have done that, but the risk would have been higher from a directed donation. I know that when many blood banks have a directed donation and the intended recipient does not need the unit, the blood bank will not use the blood for another patient, even though it has been tested and has gone through the same screening procedure as all other donations. What is the ethical duty of the blood bank with regard to directed donations?

Jonathan Moreno: Do you accept directed donation in New York? What are your ethics?

Comment from the audience: What do you do when the patient does not need it? It is discarded.

Kenrad Nelson: But you feel a duty to inform people of that option, and if you did not inform them of that option, would that not be ethical? You did not inform them that something was more dangerous, essentially.

Celso Bianco: We do, but there is conflicting information. Maybe the issue is not just the right to know, but it is the right to do something about it when you know. That is what the hemophiliacs have demanded. It is very interesting because although you gave the example of tuberculosis versus HIV, I think a slightly better example is syphilis and AIDS. New York Public

Health Law requires that when we identify an individual who is positive for syphilis, we must notify the City Department of Health within 24 hours, but we do not notify for HIV.

Jonathan Moreno: We do for AIDS.

Celso Bianco: But for HIV-positive individuals, who blood banks see far more often than AIDS patients, there is no communication. Why is it ethically acceptable not to notify (and thus not protect the partner from infection), in the case of HIV, even though notification is a legal requirement in the case of syphilis?

Jonathan Moreno: The blood bankers in my hospital in New York have said to me that they do not like autologous donation because it means there are more quantities of blood around that must be stored. They also think that it sends the wrong message because you reinforce the notion that people must protect themselves from the blood supply. That may be something like Dr. Broder's answer: I might oppose it as a matter of policy but prefer it in my own case. I cannot justify the course that New York City has decided to take except to say—with respect to HIV or AIDS informing, as well as syphilis—at this point if you are talking about contact tracing for HIV, the fact is that you are talking about hundreds of thousands of people. While it might have been a practical issue 8 or 10 years ago, I do not think anyone would find it practical anymore. It is ironic because, as many people who work with AIDS patients have said to me, when you are symptomatic, you feel like sex a lot less then when you are just infected. It does seem to turn things upside down a little bit.

Richard K. Spence: I would like to comment on the first issue that was raised. Tom Zuck mentioned that California has the Gann Act. New Jersey also has a Blood Safety Act that is an unmodified version of what California had enough good sense to change. In thinking about what I have to do in my daily practice in informed consent in terms of transfusion risk and alternatives, I see a dichotomy between what you talk about, Dr. Moreno, with hyperinforming patients, and with what Dr. Chess talked about in terms of knowing your audience, with practical implications for practice. What I find is that patients who are going to have a surgical procedure basically want to know whether they are going to get through this procedure without something harmful happening to them.

We start with whether or not they are going to need a transfusion. If I can tell them that I am going to take out their gallbladder and in my experience, they are not going to need a transfusion, they are thankful that they do not have to worry about that. However, if I am going to repair an aneurysm, they very possibly will need a transfusion. Rather than hyperinform them, because it will take a half an hour and scare them out of the room, I tell them that there are risks associated with this. They could die from the transfusion, or get an infection. These things could happen. I find that people know that because they have read about it. What they want to know is what can we do to minimize the risk. That is when we talk about autologous donation and so forth. I do not hyperinform them. I do not want to try to change their perceptions with numbers, because they know there are risks of dying, getting AIDS, whatever. There is no point arguing that getting hepatitis is more important than getting HIV from this. I find it relatively more facile for me to comply with the requirements of the law by knowing what the audience wants, listening to them, and responding to them with feedback rather than giving them a whole detailed list of what goes on.

Jonathan Moreno: I did not mean anything in particular by hyperinforming with respect to the way that the message should be communicated. I will leave that to the people who know how to communicate the message. I did not mean just throwing in the numbers, for example. I meant if there is a question about whether those people in our society would want to know about this risk, error on the side of caution and let them know about the risk, however that message is framed.

Caron Chess: Ethically, if one has an obligation to hyperinform, does that mean that there is an obligation on the part of the source to make sure that he or she is understood or only to inform, whether it is understood or not?

Jonathan Moreno: There is certainly an obligation to try to ascertain within a reasonable range of confidence and certainty whether somebody understands the information communicated or not. The question is to what extreme does one have to go, how much confidence does one have to have, and how much information does one need to be convinced that the individual understands. Those are not questions to which I have any simple answers. What we say in the clinical setting could perhaps be applied here and follows from what you just said. If people can understand the implications of what you have told them for their possible alternative futures, they can express themselves with respect to what they want for their lives, how they want to function, and that is about as much as we can expect. It probably satisfies our obligation. Obviously, we should not expect that people will be able to recite all the data in exactly the way that they have been given it in order to understand it.

Caron Chess: Various people have various needs to know. For instance, if you were the physician for an epidemiologist and you offered more information, you would probably be taken up on your offer. Someone else might never want that information. Often we think of these situations in terms of dichotomies when there are multiple options.

Jonathan Moreno: Some individuals in bioethics have suggested recently that one way to deal with the issue of how much to inform is to think of this as a tiered process of one, two, or even three tiers. For a surgical procedure, for example, you would give a relatively concise explanation, with the patient then given an explicit invitation to ask questions. If the patient asked questions, there is another tier to this information. Perhaps the third tier could even involve written material. With this tiered approach you can satisfy what most people want to know, that is, how can they get fixed, and be consistent with your moral obligations in our society to inform them, without going to an extreme.

M. Granger Morgan: I want to make three simple observations. First, there were a number of requests for prescriptive advice with respect to the issue of communication. My advice is to review studies of what people know and believe about the blood supply and the risks associated with transfusion. I would look very carefully at the quality of the methods that underlie those things. Before I could say anything much more prescriptively, I would want some empirical studies of that sort to be done. Second, I would add a warning to the advice Dr. Chess gave about going to the public health communication community. A lot of that community has not adopted the empirical style that I was talking about. If you do go to that community, be certain that you find a member who has a strong empirical commitment. Third, a comment about the role of information. Both at the individual level and certainly at the organizational level, decision making is a noisy, stochastic process influenced by many different things. For example, my carry-on bag has a lightweight smoke hood that I carry with me when I fly on airplanes. It was about a decade between the time I first learned what a smoke hood was and when I finally exerted the effort to find where they were commercially available and order one. There are a couple of other things like that I know I ought to do but have not. The point is, I would never take the second step absent the first, that is, the knowledge. Information does have an effect. It may be an effect roughly like the imposed field in Brownian motion. It is all moving around, but then the information can, in the context of all of this movement, produce a slow and perceptible drift. I would argue that telling your story repeatedly is important, even if it does not produce any obvious short-term consequence.

Question from the audience: If I understood you correctly, you place autonomy, the rights of the individual, first. How do you balance that in the national arena where we are constantly dealing with the rights of society as a whole?

Jonathan Moreno: I tried to convey my discomfort with the contemporary bioethical framework at the same time I was suggesting that it is pretty much all we have in terms of a well-developed conceptual scheme at this point. An autonomy-based ethical theory, in fact, comports pretty much with what people think about these things. The American public arguably is going to change over the years, but for the most part it does conform to the way people think about ethical issues in our society. That being the case, it is important to be sensitive to the way people think about rights as compared with communal interests. However, at the same time, we are having to be more sensitive to problems, costs, and the equitable distribution of health care services from resources that are strained.

It is not the ethicists who are going to solve the problem you have brought up. It is the fiscal realities that will drive us to find rationales within our liberal political framework that will help us to explain why what we are doing is okay. For example, we have already rationalized constraining the health care options that people have in HMO settings by saying that it is consistent with the liberal marketplace. We found a rationale base that is consistent with what we think as liberal people in the marketplace. HMOs compete and that is okay. Individual choice has to be constrained because that is the way the market works. We find ways to adapt our public philosophy to real-world constraints. However, we are not very good either in bioethical theory or in our society in figuring out how to strike the balance that you point out needs somehow to be struck.

M. Granger Morgan: Nor are we likely to be internally consistent in the way we behave. We may behave in one way much of the time in the name of efficiency but then when a particular event is identified, we behave in economic terms quite differently because we are trying, as a manner of the demonstration of our humanity or something, to make some different point. Just as decision making is a stochastic process in the context of the kinds of decisions I was talking about, policy on issues of this sort is a stochastic process. You can be absolutely certain that the one thing we will not be is consistent in the way in which we deal with all issues, nor is it even absolutely clear that we ought to be.

Jonathan Moreno: An example of how this has worked fairly successfully recently is the way that Oregon designed its health care decisions bill that finally became law. First, they asked doctors to rank procedures in terms of benefit. Then they reranked them in terms of a benefit/cost ratio analysis. They had a long list of 400 or 500 procedures, the idea being that the ones higher on the list would be funded first. Then they went to groups of people in the communities and asked them how they would rank these procedures. This step rankled a lot of health care experts because what looked like a really scientific process was now becoming infused with the irrational personal preferences of people in the community. But it proved to be a consensus builder. It is very successful and popular in Oregon. They found a way to marry these communal considerations with individual preferences and it built a consensus, convincing people that the system was responding to their wishes.

M. Granger Morgan: To recast it in multiattribute utility terms, it says that things other than efficiency matter. Equity and other concerns also count.

Question from the audience: Under most circumstances blood bankers have no contact with the recipients of the blood that they collect and manage. Instead, that communication is in the hands of others who have their own professional relationship. Do you see either any practical obligations or practical opportunities for information sharing between the blood banking community and the recipient community?

Jonathan Moreno: A few years ago this was a subject of great discussion at a meeting of the American Association of Blood Banks and there was a general agreement that that ought to happen. It seems to be needed.

Beatrice Pierce: A lot of what you have talked about in terms of trust, how that was lost and how it can be rebuilt, really strikes home to the hemophilia community. We in that community are hyperreactive now. Some want to know every little thing. Others are back to where it is all up to the physician. It is an individual process as to how much a patient wants to know, how much needs to be known, and how much is maybe just too confusing. A lot of times it is a long process to make a decision, and the amount of information that is retained in one visit can be very small. It is very important to have the avenues of communication open so that when the patient calls for the fifth time and asks a slight variation on the same question, that patient gets a very respectful answer.

Within our community a statistic of communication of HIV of one in hundreds of thousands is not real. What is real is having a friend, a family member, or someone in the community—on the average of one a week—die. So, it is biased, and it is skewed, and those skews are very hard to overcome with your statistics. When you talk about rebuilding trust, you cannot really talk about numbers. You have to talk about open communication. If you do not know, admit that you do not know. Look at the fear that is there and the fact that a lot of trust was put in physicians and the system but for various reasons those physicians and that system did not come through for their patients. You have to look at all that when you are talking about rebuilding the trust within the community. You are seeing a rebound effect as we saw with the Creutzfeldt-Jacob disease (CJD) items that have come up. Within the hemophilia community it was a knee-jerk response. Now there is something else in there to worry about. Even though we have the data indicating that CJD probably is not transmitted through plasma derivatives, we cannot forget that we have heard these reassurances before.

Celso Bianco: There is a large disassociation between what we disclose and what people get through the filters that they have. Take, for example, the question of the directed donation. We may think it is worse; therefore, we disclose to the people that it is not as safe, probably, as the autologous or the homologous transfusion. However, the people are using other filters. How do we communicate the right information? How can we convince the hemophilia community that CJD is very different from what HIV or other viruses were when all the mistrust is there? How do we turn it around?

Question from the audience: I have a question having to do with the statement that bad news has more credibility than good news and that sources of bad news are more reliable than sources of good news. I wonder what it is about our profession that has resulted in this sad state of affairs. What do we understand about the inherent cynicism in the people to whom we are speaking? How do we account for that? Do we understand something about human nature that would explain that, and if we do, short of press censorship, how can we make sure that bad news is not the news that gets all the spotlights?

Caron Chess: Based on the research that I know, it is at least Western, or American, human nature. The question is, how can you deal with the positive information you have so that people are aware of it? I think a number of different ways have been mentioned. Not withstanding the fact that I said information is not the end all and be all, people do continue to need the information. Other things have also been mentioned: the effects of physicians in dealing with their patients, the willingness to respond to questions, and the willingness to disclose information even when it may not be economically or in other ways beneficial to the source of the information.

I think that transmitting information and using the media as your primary conduit may not serve you with certain audiences. You may need to think about how you convey information or develop a dialogue with audiences who are better reached outside of the media. There is not only a responsibility to disclose information, but in terms of trust, the process of disclosure may also be important. Too often agencies go to reporters, and the people who are at risk find out about it through the media, rather than the agencies going to the local community that has a vested interest. Thus, the agencies lose trust because people ask, "Why do I have to find out about this through the newspaper?" The best way to handle disclosure is an empirical question and it needs empirical testing. The process, not just the information, is probably quite critical.

Jonathan Moreno: One strategy for rebuilding trust in your services is suggested by Theodore Lowie, a historian and political scientist. He points out that in the modern world, communities organize themselves around common characteristics that are nontraditional as a basis for community. Hemophiliacs are an interesting example. The more traditional ways of organizing are in terms of geographical proximity, ethnic or racial similarity, or perhaps class similarity. It is important for us to be aware of that fact. What would happen 2 years from now if people in the Hemophilia Foundation who are active in that community were enthusiastically supportive and confident in the blood donation system? What if they felt so much a part of what was going on and had such great confidence in what you were doing that they became ambassadors for the system? It would be quite impressive to hear people who do have routine experience be enthusiastic about the safety of the system, the openness of the professionals, and the competence of the management of these services. To take from Lowie's view, it is important in every field to know who the relevant communities are and appreciate that they may not be the ones that you would traditionally identify as a community. They may be the ones who organize themselves around characteristics that are especially important to your field, and they may be the first group with whom you forge an alliance and the first group with whom you might in fact be able to rebuild trust.

M. Granger Morgan: The previous question implied that there was something wrong with paying more attention to bad information or bad news than to good news. We know that most individuals and organizations always try to cast themselves in positive and good lights. When you do hear a bit of bad news, it tends to be a somewhat rare event, and so people tend to pay attention. Reporters are aware of this, and they use it as the vehicle to make stories more interesting. At the individual level, there is a certain underlying efficiency in paying a bit more attention to the bad news when it comes our way, as it may serve to protect us from individuals and organizations who are overly committed to their positive images.

Patients, Informed Consent, and the Health Care Team

David J. Rothman

The patient belongs inside the calculation of risk, not simply because at this point in time one really has no choice, but because it may well expand the nature of the deliberations. The patient will bring a different perspective and may help to clarify some of the choices. I will explore two cases, one of which involves trying to minimize risk and the other of which illustrates how patient involvement may have the impact of having patients live with more risk, provided that other benefits are available.

The two cases that I am going to take are, first, the model of the institutional review board (IRB), in which risk calculation is fundamental both to the origins of IRBs and to their deliberations. The second concerns the shift from radical mastectomy to lumpectomy in terms of patient involvement and risk tolerance.

Let me start with human experimentation. Until the early 1970s the calculation of risk to the subject in terms of any investigational intervention was left completely in the hands of the investigator. At the National Institutesof Health (NIH) there were some rules governing the use of normal controls. Normal controls should be informed about the research, and so forth, and there were some rudimentary comments about what the subjects should be told, but for the most part the subject was thought of as a patient. The investigator was thought of as physician, and the calculus on risks and benefits was left in the hands of a single investigator. There was really no need to collaborate with colleagues and certainly no expectation of collaborating with subjects. The investigator knew the risks, was to make a risk/benefit calculus, and proceed accordingly. By the mid-1960s this calculation of risk by the investigator alone was under attack from Beecher, Papenworth, and others.[103]

---

[103]Rothman, DJ. (1991). *Strangers at the Bedside.* New York: Basic Books.

One of the classic cases that became notorious involved Chester Southam from Cornell Medical School, New York Hospital, conducting research at the Brooklyn Jewish Chronic Disease Hospital.[104] He was interested in the body's rejection of cancer cells and thought that he could begin to solve some of the puzzles of cancer. He injected demented senile old men with foreign cancer cells. When asked why he did this without telling the subjects that he was going to be injecting them with cancer cells, he said that if he would have told them that it was cancer cells, they would have become much too frightened, would have exaggerated the risk, and would have refused to join the protocol. Because he didn't want to lose his subjects, he did not communicate to them. At one point he was asked why he didn't also inject himself, as was frequently the case with researchers. He responded that, "There aren't enough good cancer investigators." This is one of the problems of leaving it to the investigator to determine the risks.

It was decided, with NIH as the driving force, that we would no longer leave risk calculus to the investigator on the grounds that the investigator was not a neutral figure in this calculation. The investigator's first charge was to accumulate knowledge. Whether the motive was knowledge, the next grant, or the prize, investigators as a rule underestimated the risks to which they exposed their subjects.

The two major functions of the IRB are to calculate the risk-benefit ratio and ultimately to insure that the consent process is implemented in a way that those risks and benefits are clearly communicated to the subject. What we have done in the area of human experimentation is to require a collective judgment on the risk by the investigator's peers, with a few other people also involved. Equally important, the IRB insists that that finding on risk and benefit be told to the subject, so that the subject has the last word.

The difficulties, the imperfections, and the impossibility of fully informing the subject are clear and apparent. The question is how far down the disclosure of risks do you go? When consent in this process was first started in the early 1970s, you could find spoofs in the major journals. The choice of subject for the spoof was the deriding of consent by listing every risk, using circumcision as the test case.

In the end, we now require communication about risk to the subject, and we are going about it in a very decentralized way, leaving it to local IRBs, and to individual patients to calculate the nature of how much risk should be taken.

Were Creutzfeldt-Jakob disease part and parcel of an experimental protocol, knowing what we know now, would that risk be communicated to the subject? The answer to that would really depend ultimately on individual

---

[104]*Ibid*, pp 77–93.

IRBs. They might bend over backwards in an experimental protocol and say, "Yes, that ought to be included." They probably would not rule out an experiment simply on the basis of that unknown risk being present, but they might. The key point is that they certainly would want the subject ultimately to make the decision about the risk.

You are not going to find an existing national body that is going to make that decision on its own. You will find in elements of risk calculus that we have accepted informed consent as the basis for approval. We anticipate through IRB and consent that ultimately we do share risk analysis collectively and ultimately trust the choice made by the subject. We now tend on the whole in human experimentation to be risk minimizing. In the area of research communication of risk, sharing information about risk, and calculating risk against benefit is not merely standard, it is mandated, and however imperfect in practice, it is altogether the requirement.

If you look at the clinical setting and allow me my choice of the case of radical mastectomy versus lumpectomy, you begin to find a second and very interesting model in terms of risk calculus. The decision in favor of radical mastectomy as almost the only procedure to be used in all cases of breast cancer lasted well into the late 1970s and even into the early 1980s. The ultimate reason was the surgeon's response of risk minimization. The shift from radical mastectomy to lumpectomy is complicated. Parts of the story involve radiology and oncology, as well as psychiatry. No roster of participants who moved us from mastectomy to lumpectomy would be complete without talking about women and patients' groups themselves. It would not be an exaggeration to say that although the change certainly was abetted, encouraged, and finally conclusively established in the territory of medicine, the role of women activists was absolutely critical.

There the risk calculus shifted the other way as opposed to the psychological pains and physical pains of a radical mastectomy. Where the choice turned out to be a realistic one, many women prepared to carry the additional burden of risk in return for the benefit of not undergoing radical mastectomy.

That conversation between a surgeon or oncologist and woman patient is as complicated a conversation medically and emotionally speaking as one can imagine. The variables that go into the risks of each procedure are very exquisite. It is very difficult, intellectually and emotionally, to parse out the risks, and yet it is being done all the time. In this day and age for a breast surgeon in this country to say, as I recently heard from a physician in Israel, "This is much too complicated, I am simply going to make the decision and not involve the woman," would be absurd. It may well be than an older patient or a patient overwhelmed by the diagnosis may turn to her surgeon and say, "I don't want to hear about it. Do what you want to do." That certainly happens. The right to say no to information certainly is to be respected, but the standard is surely to share the information about risk, although it is complicated. In the area of clinical practice, we have clearly reached the point where sharing the decision-making about risk after intensive conversation is standard.

It is fairly apparent that clinically many physicians have great difficulty communicating risks to their patients. Some are paternalistic. Physicians on the whole do not do a very good job communicating about risk. There is a fear that if they tell a patient all the risks, the patient won't be compliant. Physicians may also be trying to be protective of patients by trying not to worry them. It seems if you tell the patient there is a side effect, that patient will call you tomorrow and report the side effect.

In summary, it is easy to spoof risk disclosure and point to the flaws, but I would suggest on the basis of my two models that the benefits of doing it far outweigh whatever the problems are. Furthermore, physicians probably don't have a lot of choice any longer. In experimentation, they certainly don't. Dealing with women and breast cancer, they don't. The list is going to get longer, not shorter. You may agree or disagree with one or another of my arguments, but in the end it is moving in exactly the direction I have described.

DISCUSSION

Paul Russell: There is no question that we must strive toward informed consent. There is also no doubt that it is a very flawed process and that we cannot get to total informed consent. Our responsibility lies with the issue of diminishing risks as you get out toward the end of the risk curve. It is difficult, but it is an important thing to do. I am concerned about it. How far should I go in telling people about risks?

David Rothman: In an experimental setting, I would think you would want to go further. In a therapeutic setting, the patient gives you cues. I am sure older patients, or maybe those less educated, might press you less.

Paul Russell: I go as far as the patient wants to go.

David Rothman: You are not going to bludgeon the patient with information, but if the patient is a long-distance runner and there is a 5 percent risk that this surgery is going to keep him off the track for the rest of his life, you might well want to tell him that. If the patient that comes in is rather corpulent, beer drinking, and poker playing, the 5 percent risk to a running career would be irrelevant. You will tailor it. You are going to go down the major items and then, depending on that patient's tolerance for information, you go down below the normal list to include those that you think would be particularly relevant for the patient.

Paul Russell: I think that is a helpful guide, but it doesn't get me all the way.

Edward A. Dauer: In those instances in which a patient's perception or evaluation of a risk is not consonant with its actual quantity, is it the physician's responsibility to respect the patient's evaluation as it is or to try to correct that perception and bring it back into line with the actual quantification?

David Rothman: The answer to that is absolutely yes, you have to bring it back into line. No patient is going to ever get to exercise informed consent on his own unless the physician helps him realize it. You have to correct. A patient may have a fear that is completely out of perspective. You will give the information. What do you then do when a patient still says, "No thank you"? You try a second time, but it may not be appropriate to try the fifth time. That you must make an effort is absolutely clear, but in the end when you are content that that patient has understood you, then it remains the patient's choice.

Llewellys Barker: By telling patients what the risks are, the practical approach is very appropriate. I have been on both sides of this process. In your mind, does what we tell patients the risks are equate with "these are the risks we tolerate"?

David Rothman: I have a lot of trouble with "we." Is that the five people who are sitting in the lab or the five people at an NIH consensus conference? I might prefer "we" to become "I." The point of my remarks is to personalize it, individualize it, and communicate it. The "we tolerate" formulation may make it too easy not to communicate.

Communication of Risk and Uncertainty to Patients

Donald Colburn

I wear a lot of hats in the world of hemophilia. I have hemophilia, severe Factor VIII deficiency. I also have HIV disease, and I happen to be president and chief executive officer of American Homecare Federation, which is a company that provides service to people with hemophilia. In addition, I am currently serving as a member of the National Hemophilia Foundation's (NHF) Blood Products Monitoring Committee, and I am chairing the legislative campaign for passage of the Ricky Ray Relief Act.

I am going to discuss the general concept of blood safety and take a look at how we currently educate folks. Having been on the receiving end of that education, I would say that I have not experienced the inclusion of the patient in decision making that you have discussed. The attitude of the physicians is still, "Do what I say. This is good for you. If you don't do it, you will be more ill."

With respect to blood and blood products, I believe we should be moving toward a signed informed consent. We can certainly talk about how far we go in levels of exploring uncertain risks. Unfortunately, the process of sharing the information necessary to institute informed consent is time-consuming, and, as we know, the health care system is already operating with a lack of quality time spent with patients. The challenge we have is to devise a mechanism that will allow blood bankers, for instance, who are very interested in blood safety issues to serve a broader role in the process of educating patients.

There has been a great deal of discussion about the pamphlet that is put out by American ssociation of Blood Banks (AABB) in conjunction with the Council of Community Blood Centers (CCBC) and the Red Cross. Designed for recipients of cellular blood products, it is supposed to mimic a package insert as far as information. To date I have not found one person with hemophilia or another condition who received this pamphlet at the time of receiving a cellular product. Even that mechanism isn't being utilized. What can we do that will allow some "right of information" for that patient? For starters, we can provide signed and informed consent with chronic users of blood products on an annualized basis.

In addition, we first must make information understandable for people with various levels of education. The second thing that we have to do is to present the information in an unbiased manner. Then we have to be certain that patient is up to date with the information when he makes that decision. Once there has been uncertainty about a particular product, that uncertainty hinders communication even more, as we experienced with HIV. The patient, as the blood products' consumer, should have the ultimate role in the decision. Without that type of participation, without informed consent that somebody has on file somewhere, then the whole thing becomes bogus if a disease is transmitted.

To sum up, it is important, tremendously important, that we present materials to people in an unbiased fashion that they can understand. One would like to think that the patient would have many more questions, especially in a situation involving chronic use. As far as communicating the risk of uncertainty, that is a tough one. Blood goes through various processes which eradicate most diseases most of the time. However, there are many conditions that are not tested for and that we don't know about. Those are unknown risks. It is important that we don't panic the person, but that he or she understands that there will always be risks in any medication. Even recombinant products have a risk factor. That is part of life. We have to make a sincere effort to bring the patient into the loop, and in some areas it works very well. It works really well in discussion groups like this, but when you get back out into the field you often hear remarks from folks like, "Doc just said that this is what I should do," remarks which reinforce the continuing absence of shared information and informed consent. At NHF we are working very hard to empower our consumers to come back to the medical community with a lot of questions. We think it is important. We have had a very severe lesson as a result of our own complacency.

DISCUSSION

Paul Russell: Having the patient specifically sign makes a lot of sense, and that is really pretty much what we are trying to do throughout. In the case of transfusion it could be applied a little bit more broadly and repeatedly in the case of patients like those you are familiar with.

Harvey Klein: Informed consent for blood transfusion has been national policy since 1986. I don't know whether that is standard of care in the outside world and whether every institution practices that, but the AABB, for example, has had that written form widely disseminated to every one of its members since 1986. The circular of information, the so-called package insert, was not really developed for patient use any more than the package inserts in the drugs that you get. The package inserts were developed to inform the physicians, whose job it is to inform the patient who receives a blood transfusion.

Paul Schmidt: There was a study about 3 years ago in which a group of investigators doing informed consent talked to patients after surgery and then some months later. The patients didn't remember what had been discussed and their understanding was different.

Donald Colburn: You are always going to have that obstacle. My emphasis is on the chronic user of medical services. There the time is importantly spent because that patient is going to take up a lot of the medical services' time. The better informed that person is, the better the relationship will be. The difficulty that we have observed in the hemophilia community is that when there is a perception that there has not been the opportunity to participate in the therapeutic regimen decision, then all the other systems become distrusted. That perceived breach by the individual causes a great deal of harm, even if the patient would not have remembered everything he or she was told.

Henrik Bendixen: The point is that informed consent is not a freestanding event but should be part of the continuum of interaction between physician and patient.

David Rothman: The world wide web on the Internet is becoming a real player. A colleague of ours talked about the fact that his patients ask where the newest protocol is. The AIDS community brought us into that consumer-based knowledge concerning protocol availability. If you don't have a protocol going they are not coming to your institution. Although I know those stories about how if you poll the patient 3 months later he doesn't remember the consent form, there are lots of newer stories about patient groups that are all on the Internet communicating with each other in terms of where the best protocol is.

Harold Sox: At Dartmouth there has been a reverse epidemic of operations for benign prostatic hypertrophy as a result of Wennberg and Mulley's work.[105] They developed video disks that convey in an individualized way

---

[105] Kasper, JF, AG Mulley Jr, JE Wennberg (1992). Developing shared decision-making programs to improve the quality of health care (comments). *Quality Review Bulletin, 18(6):* 183–190.

the risks and benefits of a procedure with respect to the various therapeutic options. As a result patients bring a lot more information to the discussion with the physician. The process of the discussion is at least enlightened and may be even truncated somewhat. This might be another instance in which annual provision of informed consent might be in order.

James Reilly: Whether we are a blood center providing blood to the transfusion center or a product manufacturer providing products to a treatment facility, where in your view is the communication breakdown? Is it that we are not providing enough to the physician or that the physician is not communicating to the patient?

Donald Colburn: I did ask a number of blood bankers why isn't that circular used, for instance, because it is supposed to go up with every unit. I started to probe in that direction and the responses I got were amazing. "When we first got them we started sending them up, and all of a sudden I got calls from about five or six different hematologists. 'What the hell are you sending up to my patients? If I want them to know anything, I will tell them.'" The overall problem is in physician communication to patient. I see it as time management because it takes a long time to be certain someone is educated.

Frederick Manning: One of the projects I have been involved in here at the Institute of Medicine involved an experimental drug and the whole question of informed consent: how much is enough; how much should you tell the patients. It turned out the drug did not work out all that well. There was a lot of talk from patients about what they should have been told. In the process we did a little poll of the committee, who were all relatively eminent clinical researchers. The question was whether they could recall in their careers ever having a potential subject in one of their experiments who listened to their pitch, read the informed consent form, and said, "No, I am not interested." In fact, none of them could think of a single instance in which that happened. For the audience today, I would ask you to think back and tell us how many times have you had a patient leave the office after you described what the risks were? Maybe there are some inherent limitations about how scared you can make a patient who has already come to you and decided that he or she is going to trust you.

Paul Russell: I have certainly had patients decide against surgery after I explained the risks. We have immensely complicated clinical protocols that have to be applied to almost every patient we see. When they come in for an organ transplant they may have to sign about half a dozen consent forms. It is not uncommon to have one or two of them be inappropriate. Their refusal may not be because they are scared, but because it is an immensely complicated setting. I think you are thinking of a setting with a simple, straightforward, single question. In the situations that I deal with, there is an awful lot of experimentation of all kinds, one superimposed on top of another. There are patients who are in several protocols at once.

David Rothman: There are protocols out there that don't get to enroll patients. There will be a research team to which the treating physician may or may not dispatch his or her patient. For example, at our institution the investigator who really wants to figure out if bone marrow transplantation has any efficacy in breast cancer cannot get patients to enroll because if you want it, it is out there to be had, and if you don't want it, you are not going to leave yourself to a random draw. No one goes into the protocol.

Elaine Eyster: There are two very different types of protocols. One is the type that has been referred to, in which we have a variety of experimental studies for persons who are infected with HIV. We present those and patients may or may not choose to go on that protocol. It doesn't interfere with our relationship with them, but they have that choice. On the other hand, we have a routine informed consent that everybody signs and re-signs on some sort of interim basis saying that they agree to participate in a study in which their blood can be used for certain purposes. Most patients will accept that as part of what we do, but others will say, "No, I don't care to do that." That wish is honored, and they are not included in whatever study that you are doing.

William Sherwood: There is also a great deal of informed consent that is really for comfort. Virtually all hospitals instituted an informed consent for transfusion, particularly prior to surgery. There are a couple of paragraphs given to the patient at a time when that patient has a lot of other things to sign, and the patient is under a good deal of stress having surgery the next day or the next morning. What we are searching for is just how far to go with informed consent. An interplay with the patient to try to find out how far to go was suggested, but I had trouble with that. I would like to be more uniform. I would like to be able to tell all patients what the potentials are and what I should be doing. Is there a way to stratify these risks—proven, potential, and theoretical—and where should we draw those lines? It is difficult to handpick something for each patient when you know in the long run that the patient will be disaffected in some way and later come back and say, "Why didn't you tell me about that risk?" I cannot come back and say to them, "I didn't think you needed to know it." We need more guidance on how deep to go in the risk spectrum in helping patients understand.

David Rothman: When an institutional review board (IRB) does a risk assessment for informed consent, it lists the major potential side effects by percentage; it keeps going down to maybe include some in the 10 percent range, but it probably doesn't go down to the 1 percent range. I don't know that all the patients read it, but they are going to certainly read the major untoward effects. The kinds of complaints that often end up being told to me are one in which the patient has been given a prescription, but the ordinary side effect was not mentioned to the patient. The patient experiences it, calls the physician the next day, and physician says, "Relax, it is one of the side effects," to which the response is, "So, why didn't you tell me?" We need to be between the extremes of parsing it out to 1 percent and telling a patient, "Look, you are going to be taking this. Here are the major side effects."

Donald Colburn: I have signed off on admission to a hospital on a blood form. What you sign is incredible. If you sit there and challenge the document, you become a troublesome patient at that point. If you say, "I don't understand this," the person who is doing the intake to put you into the hospital is a clerk for the most part and responds, "Sign these forms." You ask "What happens if I don't sign them?" and the clerk says "We cannot put you in the hospital." You sign the forms. There is some degree of pressure that is put on the patient at that stage, in addition to whatever else may have been tried to have been communicated.

Harvey Klein: Many good hospitals don't consider informed consent a form given at the time of intake with a clerk. That really isn't informed consent.

David Rothman: Exactly. What could be a worse time? We have some data on hospitals trying to do advanced directives at the time of admission. Could there be a worse time to do anything, especially because somebody knows you are coming.

James Allen: When you talk about listing potential adverse side effects in the 10 percent range, but not the 1 percent range, is that a 10 percent risk of occurrence versus a 1 percent risk of occurrence? Surely, for serious effects such as risk of HIV infection post-transfusion, a risk of one in several tens of thousands is considered highly significant and certainly a "must notify."

David Rothman: You are absolutely right.

VI

No-Fault Insurance

Administrative and "No-Fault" Systems for Compensating Medically Related Injuries

Edward A. Dauer

A committee of the Institute of Medicine (IOM) that has been examining the history of HIV and the blood supply recently issued a report which included among its several recommendations the suggestion that "The federal government should consider establishing a no-fault compensation system for individuals who suffer adverse consequences from the use of blood or blood products."[106] Unlike first-party no-fault insurance, a no-fault compensation system is a complex and in many ways controversial idea. In the special setting of medical practice injury such as infections associated with blood transfusions, it is particularly interesting—though in some quarters of the legal profession no less controversial.

The IOM's recommendation came without discussion, so far as I can tell from reading the report, but it is not an unwelcome idea. There has already been quite a bit of activity in that area, including a soon-to-be-implemented experiment in blood banking itself. Before addressing that program, however, and other particular examples, I would like to begin with an overview of what no-fault compensation programs are about and why they may be of interest to us.

No-fault programs are systems for compensating people who have been injured, and are offered (or required) in lieu of or as alternatives to the conventional civil liability system. They are designed principally to respond to certain diseconomies that many believe are endemic to the legal system as it currently exists. To help you appreciate this more graphically, I would like to share with you a chapter of the cultural history of American civil liability law. It is a story which I believe was first recounted by Charles Lamb 200 years ago in his *Essays of Elia*.

---

[106]Institute of Medicine (1995). *HIV and the Blood Supply: An Analysis of Crisis Decisionmaking.* Washington, D.C.: National Academy Press.

At one time in early human history people ate food without cooking it. They would gather fruits and vegetables and eat them just as they found them. Every now and then they would venture into the forest where they might find an animal, usually a small pig, which they might capture and kill. They discovered that eating these animals freshly killed was not very tasty, and, they slowly realized that it had some adverse health effects. One day there began by accident a ferocious forest fire that roared through the surrounding woods, destroying tens of thousands of acres and all of the creatures that had lived there. When the fire was finally out, the people wandered into the charred woods and saw that as a consequence of the fire some of the wild pigs had been roasted. They tasted them, and found them to be much tastier than they were before. There also seemed to be fewer of the adverse health effects. From that day forward it therefore came to be that whenever someone had a yen for barbecued pig, they would start a forest fire. Thus, the original efficiency model for the American litigation system.

The formal litigation system is an adversarial process that generates decisions by nonexpert fact finders. It has essentially five jobs to do, each of them very labor intensive. One of the jobs is to investigate the facts of the incident, to assess "causation," i.e., did the injuries and consequences complained of flow from the error or omission alleged? Second, and more or less simultaneously with determining causation, the legal system investigates the relevant history both to determine what happened and to characterize what happened by comparing it with the relevant standards concerning what *should* have happened. If the historical behavior did not meet the required standard, it can be labeled as having been "negligent," and thus the defendants are determined to have been at "fault." This too is a very labor-intensive investigation.

Third, if both negligence and causation are found, there is another investigation of the facts about the injury and a prediction about the future, to determine the measure of what we call damages. This is the gross amount that the plaintiff will recover from the defendant. It is in fact a best guess about a future of medical care and disability losses that is, in the conventional trial, never tested by the reality of that future.

In particularly egregious cases there is a larger social function, in which the legal system considers the possibility of punishing the parties at fault and deterring such faulty actions by them and others like them through the imposition of punitive damages. This requires yet another set of investigations, calculations, and measurements.

The legal system's fifth task, in addition to all of the preceding, is to administer the forum and the mechanisms by which people who do not want to cooperate in addressing the matter or who do not want to share the necessary information can be forced to do so. And it provides the arena in which all of these functions are managed. These five are the outputs—these are what the litigation process does. These jobs and their counterparts in a no-fault system can be summarized in a simple table (Table 8).

TABLE 8 Functions of Litigation and No-Fault Systems

Litigation	No-Fault System
Through an adversarial process, presided over by a nonexpert fact finder	Through a process that is more administrative than adversarial and that is managed by experts,
1. Investigates the facts of the incident, to assess "causation."	1. Investigates causation or, for certain injuries, presumes it.
2. Determines the relevant standards, to establish "negligence."	
3. Investigates the facts of the injury and predicts the future to determine the measure of "damages."	3. Finds damages from a table of injuries or on an as-incurred basis.
4. Considers the possibility of punishment through "punitive damages."	
5. Provides the forum and the mechanism to require disclosure of information and to enforce the result.	5. Typically establishes nonlitigation system to handle disputes; disclosure of information by agreement.

No-fault systems look very different. They are typically (though not always) administrative rather than adversarial. They are usually managed (and the decisions are made by) people who are expert in the specific problems being reviewed. They do less than litigation does.

In a no-fault system causation is retained. The question is, "Did this action cause that damage?" If the answer is yes, the next step is to calculate the compensation, which in some systems (such as workers' compensation) is done by looking them up in a table of injuries rather than by doing individualized adjudications. While such "scheduled benefits" are not highly individualized, the process is certainly more efficient. A second source of efficiency is the "pay-as-you-go" approach, in which rather than awarding the claimant a sum based on a once-for-always guess about the future, the system may elect to pay for medical care and disability losses if, as, and when they arise. Increased accuracy can be achieved this way, and thus a higher degree of efficiency in the application of the available compensation funds.

Finally, as to the fifth job, in many no-fault systems the exchange of information is done by consent rather than by decree, and the enforcement of this exchange can be achieved in whatever way is necessary.

The ambition of a no-fault system is in large part to eliminate litigation's enormous processing costs by eliminating some of the most labor-intensive aspects of what litigation generally does. We learned, for example, as we were litigating asbestos injuries that only about 40 cents of each dollar spent in litigation went to compensate the plaintiffs; the other 60 cents went to overhead. Administrative systems, by contrast, generally operate with a 9 or 10 or sometimes 20 percent overhead ratio. Thus, in an appropriate setting, one-half to two-thirds of the operating costs can be saved by eliminating some of the jobs done by litigation.

A no-fault system does other things as well. It decouples the right of compensation from the determination of medical error. The negligence system puts those two together, saying that unless the physician or health care provider made a negligent mistake, this injured person gets nothing. If there was a negligent mistake, this other person gets paid. It is charged, at least, that this linkage results in "defensive medicine" as often as it results in effective deterrence, another inefficiency in the process. Table 9 summarizes some of the other characteristics of no-fault systems and litigation, again as seen by an observer who is an acknowledged fan of the concept. Perhaps needless to say, not every trial lawyer would agree with this way of displaying the comparison.

There are a number of distinctions between litigation and no-fault or administrative systems. One is that in litigation the amount of compensation is a prediction not corrected by the later reality. In most trials, you only go to court once. Juries will tend to overcompensate injured plaintiffs because they do not know what is going to happen to them in the future. In an administrative system, properly structured, compensation can be triggered by actual needs as they occur, and therefore, the efficiency of expenditures can be higher.

Litigation is also highly disruptive and creates a daily drumbeat of news that is seldom very productive. On the other hand, the public nature of litigation sometimes has advantages. No-fault systems, when they operate privately, may not reveal for public scrutiny errors, problems, and questions that would in fact be revealed and investigated publicly if they were grist for the mills of the courts. There is a trade-off to be considered there.

However, litigation analyzes medical questions in an adversarial setting rather than in a scientific setting. No-fault systems typically use expert decision makers rather than the lay juries of the legal forum, and may gain some accuracy if not authenticity with respect to issues such as causation in trying to reach its adjudications.

TABLE 9 Selected Characteristics of Litigation and No-Fault Systems

Litigation	No-Fault System
Quantum of compensation is a prediction, not later corrected.	Compensation can be limited and focused.
Process is inefficient, public, and disruptive.	Process is more efficient, but there is less public scrutiny.
Analyzes medical and scientific questions in an adversarial rather than scientific venue.	Can use expert decision makers as to relevant issues.
Compensates far fewer than the number injured—negligently or not.	Will compensate many more than a fault-based system.
(Over)compensates some who have no compensable claim.	Claims severity declines, but claims frequency rises.
Linkage to deterrence and quality of care is uncertain.	Linkage to patient safety systems is different.
Adverse public and professional effects encourage "defensive" behaviors.	Deterrence may be intact, since the relationship between costs and errors is more accurate.

In addition, litigation makes two kinds of errors. First, the number of people who are negligently injured and who are compensated through the tort system is the minority. Most negligently injured people are not compensated by the tort system at all. On the other hand, about half of the people who do recover damages from the tort system shouldn't have, if measured by the standard of negligence. The reason for this is that the process allows for bargaining: "I won't sue you if you give me X dollars." Thus, we end up with both kinds of errors at the same time—undercompensation through the cost-barriers to meritorious claims and overcompensation through the nuisance potential of nonmeritorious claims. This also helps to make the efficiency of compensation very low, and particularly so in medical injury cases.

When we shift to a no-fault system, the number of people who are compensated rises. We get many more claims than the fault-based system does. Analysts refer to this as an increase in "frequency." However, average claims "severity" tends to decline, and thus, the net indemnity cost—what we pay for compensation—may not actually rise at all. The savings devoted to paying more claims come from the reduction in the number and size of "outlier" awards and in the reduction in the costs of processing.

With respect again to litigation and the linkage between liability and deterrence, the question is whether doctors behave better if they are concerned with being sued. The evidence is quite doubtful. One of the things that we do know is that fault-based liability tends to distort behavior as the practitioners become concerned with doing things that will help to win later lawsuits as well as things that will help to avoid errors. Patient safety may not be enhanced by fault-based liability as much as by, in effect, strict liability.[107] A no-fault system sharpens the deterrent effect, it has been argued, rather than removing it, as the practitioners now become *responsible* for all adverse outcomes caused by their acts rather than being *liable* for only those adverse outcomes that are capable of being proven negligent. Thus, I am not convinced that we will reduce patient safety if we move away from fault-based liability.

In no-fault systems the linkage between patient safety and compensation is deliberately undone. Patient safety can then be examined through devices that the medical establishment thinks are appropriate, while compensation is taken care of independently of that. No-fault systems can be created in any of a number of ways, as Table 10 suggests.

One way is by statute, of which an example is the National Vaccine Program. Virginia and Florida have statutory no-fault systems that pay compensation in cases of neurological injuries to neonates. The federal Black Lung Program for miners is also a no-fault system. Worker's Compensation is probably the best and the most common example, and an example of a process—even with all of its much-heralded flaws—that operates on a cost ratio of 20 percent or so, compared with the tort system's 50+ percent. Several European countries have made payments to hemophilia patients infected with HIV through Factor VIII, either through legal enactment or simply because they are all part of the public health system. These examples tend to be quasiadjudicative systems that operate on the basis of schedules of benefits. They are very focused, limited applications. Typically, negligence is irrelevant.

---

[107]There is a considerable economic literature on this subject, much of it stemming from the work of Ronald Coase and others, who have argued that in a transaction cost-free world, the rule of liability does not matter. Unfortunately, the world is not transaction cost-free.

TABLE 10 Some Types and Examples of No-Fault and Administrative Systems

Types	Examples
Statutory	National Vaccine Program, Virginia and Florida Neurological Birth Injury, Miners' Black Lung, Workers' Compensation, European Hemophilia Payments (ex gratia or through public health financing system), Utah and Colorado Initiatives *Quasiadjudicative systems, tables of benefits, very limited applications. Negligence is typically irrelevant.*
Judicial	Dalkon shield, Agent Orange, DDT, milk-borne *Salmonella*, Asbestos *Arise typically in mass disasters; born from class actions or bankruptcy plans; usually follow a period of intense litigation.*
Contractual	High school sports injury insurance and other private arrangements *Typically avoid public litigation; may or may not address fault; some use tables of benefits.*

There is a second form of no-fault that occurs in cases of mass or serial injuries from a single product or event, usually after a period of intense litigation through which the participants have figured out, by living through the early cases, where the later cases are likely to come out if they go to court. The early cases, to be candid about it, set the "market values" around which the later cases can be more efficiently settled. These are no-fault in the sense that they are class settlements in which the issue of fault is by agreement made irrelevant to individual cases. Some examples are the Dalkon shield, Agent Orange, two incidents involving DDT, and some asbestos cases. What happens in these judicial examples is that eventually the combatants realize that the amount of money spent to litigate later cases is being wasted—that there is a certain amount of money that is either going to go to the claimants or to the lawyers. Thus, we have examples of product-specific no-fault programs emerging from the courts and some from judicially approved settlements of class actions.

There are, in addition, some contractual, private programs. These are not arbitration programs, like Kaiser's, in which negligence is still relevant, even though the change in the forum may be quite radical. These are programs in which the sponsor has determined that it will pay for all losses caused by its acts, without regard to the legal standard of care. The high school sports injury program is one in which a guarantee is made that if a high school athlete is injured while playing football or other sports, an insurance policy arranged for by the school system pays his actual medical and disability costs, without regard to negligence and in lieu of an action in the courts. This occurs not by operation of law but simply by private contract.

There is an advantage to embracing no-fault by contract, as well as a number of disadvantages. This, however, can better be examined in the context of some specific kinds of programs rather than by way of a general overview.

The Colorado and Utah Models of Compensating Patient Injury

Mason Howard

I am going to describe what is happening simultaneously in Utah and Colorado, aiming toward legislative creation of a sole-remedy administrative system for compensating patient injury. This effort comes from looking at our own experience in Colorado and also looking at the work of the Harvard Public Health School commissioned by the state of New York and published in 1990 under the title of *Patients, Doctors and Lawyers, Patient Injury Compensation Malpractice Litigation*.

The Harvard Public Health School study demonstrated that the inpatient injury rate, as documented from the hospital record, was 4 percent in the state of New York in 1984. About one-quarter of those were due to provider negligence that was also documented in the medical record.

People have taken this number and used it variously. Some public interest groups have advertised that we kill more people in hospitals than we do on the highways. I am not sure that is an accurate reflection of what that study says, but a 4 percent injury rate and a 1 percent negligence rate is not a goal we ought to be striving for. I think we ought to be looking at something better than that.

What they did in New York was to compare the documented injuries in the medical record with the litigation files in that state for 1984. They found that of the people who were injured with no demonstrable negligence, only 10 percent ever made any monetary recovery from the court system, and of those who were injured with documentable negligence in the record, only 20 percent made a monetary recovery. Overall, of all the people and records studied, only 15 percent made some kind of recovery. The results speak to the vast cost and inefficiency of the system.

If we talk in Colorado to the licensure authorities of the health care system, it is the feeling of the people who operate these programs that through all the mechanisms that are now available we find about one-third of the substandard medical practice that is going on in Colorado. That includes malpractice litigation, patient complaints, hospital disciplinary actions, and so forth. Thus, two-thirds of the substandard medical practice that is occurring goes undiscovered. In Colorado in 1995, we will collect $47 million from the 75 percent of the physicians who must buy insurance.

In Colorado we have the classic tort reforms that have occupied the last 20 years of state legislative activity with $1 million cap on recoveries, including noneconomic damages. Although we have the best tort reforms in the country, it still costs 4,000 doctors $47 million to fund their malpractice.

In the New York study, the Harvard estimate was that in a year in which the providers paid $1.2 billion in premiums for their liability insurance, it would have cost about $900 million to pay all of the people who were projected to have been injured in that state in that year. That leaves enough of a cushion, if those numbers are anywhere nearly accurate, to run the system on the basis that most state workers' compensation companies run, which is with about a 20 percent overhead.

The system that we envision and that we hope will become a sole remedy for compensating medical injury in the state of Colorado will be three pronged. The first thing that will occur is a very simplified one-page application process on the part of the patient: "I, John Doe, think I was hurt by this medical person on this date in this facility."

Mandated provider reporting of the injury will produce this patient complaint. This will lead to three things: first, compensation of the patient on a net out-of-pocket cost basis; second, an enhanced system of provider discipline; and, third, risk management not oriented toward avoiding successful malpractice litigation but oriented toward avoiding injury.

Compensation would include net out-of-pocket costs, lost wages, future health care costs, rehabilitation, and possibly household production. No compensation system currently addresses this issue of lost but previously unpaid household production. That may be difficult, particularly if we look at the potential costs, which may blow the affordability of such a system right out of the water and make it unworkable.

We are not adequately disciplining physicians. One of the reasons is that we have such a terrible system of finding the problem. As I mentioned earlier, the licensure authorities believe they find about one-third of the things that happen through any of the various existing reporting mechanisms. Our system provides the potential for a 100 percent screen if we assume that we can get 100 percent of the people who sustain an injury to report it and/or have their providers report it. In the proposed system every complaint would be investigated and the results would automatically be forwarded to the licensing authority.

It is important to keep investigation as an element of this for two reasons. First, it is a societal issue that improves the system that we have, and second, it retains the possibility of the deterrent effect that is found in the tort system.

By creating a central database that is based on 100 percent of screened injuries by location and provider, this system allows risk management efforts to focus on improving the quality of medical care rather than simply avoiding successful malpractice litigation.

We believe, based on the work done in New York by the Harvard School of Public Health, that there are already enough premium dollars in Colorado to fund this system if we take out the litigation costs that in Colorado now consume about 50 cents of every premium dollar. Then the providers themselves can provide enough funding for this that it covers both the indemnity costs and the operational costs.

We now do a very good job of experience rating physicians on a specialty-oriented basis. It could be even better if we knew about all the injuries that occur in the state. At some point, if this system is good enough, we may be able to request that the state provide some of the costs through the general fund.

The plan both in Colorado and in Utah was to do a study very similar to what was done in New York, and that study has been done. After the data are compiled and readied for analysis, we will create legislation appropriate to our state, begin to educate our legislature through the session in 1996 and the study sessions in the summer of 1996, and then introduce legislation in the first week of January 1997. Our odds of success are only 50/50 at best because this is a pretty revolutionary idea and is not happening anywhere else. I'll close at this point with a quick summary of the major features of the proposal:

• Administrative no-fault system created by legislation (target date: 1997 session).
• Exclusive remedy for all cases of medical injury and accident (definitions to exclude expected but disappointing outcomes being studied).
• Compensation for economic losses including disability beyond a waiting period. Medical payments are in excess of underlying health insurance. Includes survivor benefits.
• Improved provider discipline through enhanced reporting and mandatory risk management focused on more collected data. Providers must self-report incidents and notify patients of the system.
• The administrative agency will both manage the compensation system and, separately, investigate incidents and errors.
• Initial funding will be by provider payments to the agency equal to their previous insurance payments. Thereafter, payments will be based on experience rating.

DISCUSSION

Edward A. Dauer: A group of attorneys, blood bankers, hospital administrators and claims executives, and others have been working over the past 2 years to develop a pilot project to test the feasibility of no-fault compensation for blood- and transfusion-related injuries. The program, which was initiated by the American Asociation of Blood Banks (AABB), the Council of Community Blood Centers (CCBC), and the American Red Cross (ARC) working in concert, differs in some significant ways from the programs just described that are being readied for testing in Colorado and Utah. One significant difference is that the Colorado and Utah experiments both require legislation. The AABB-CCBC-ARC program does not; it is entirely private.

The origin of this private model was the aftermath of the transfusion-related HIV tragedy of the early 1980s. Having experienced the difficulties of the associated litigation, in addition to the personal and organizational stresses of the episodes, the leadership of the three blood banking organizations decided that they would like to have some alternative in place for the future, should there ever be another such threat to the safety of the blood supply. They commissioned the Center for Public Resources (CPR) to examine the possibilities. One of the suggestions made by CPR in its report to the sponsors was that they explore more fully a privately run no-fault system, limited to transfusion-related injuries, to serve the needs of the blood banking community and—because it would thus be attractive to potential hospital and physician participants—to act as a demonstration model for medical injuries generally. The sponsors accepted the proposal and determined that a pilot program should be implemented.

The model is being developed as a pilot program, for initial implementation in a single state. There are two dominant blood suppliers in that state, making the organizational tasks relatively straightforward. The leadership of both were positive toward examining the possibilities. In addition, the medical community was particularly sophisticated about alternative dispute resolution (ADR) as a result of their own experience with legislative efforts, and the political system appeared to be more accessible than would be true in a much larger state. A working group was assembled under the leadership of the state hospital association, and the hospital community responded eagerly to the invitation to participate in the study.

The outline of the no-fault model is provided in Table 11. It will cover designated transfusion-associated injuries, including all blood-borne pathogens, transfusion errors, donor injuries, and other designated incidents. When an individual incurs a covered injury, the group of participating organizations, including the implicated hospitals, blood banks, physicians, and their insurers, will make an offer to the plaintiff to compensate him or her for economic losses on a no-fault basis. The offer is made after the injury (as opposed to a contract entered into with the patient in advance) and will address that person's disability and medical needs attributable to the medical injury as they arise.

TABLE 11 Elements of the Transfusion-Related Injury Compensation Program

1. The program will be a *pilot*, with no certain termination date, subscribed to by blood centers, participating hospitals, and physicians and their insurers,

2. that offers to persons with *designated transfusion-associated injuries*—all blood-borne pathogens and transfusion errors—*after the injury occurred*,

3. compensation for attributable economic losses, including *actual medical costs if and when incurred and* (subject to some limits) actual disability wage losses,

4. on a *non-fault* basis, but only for injuries actually *caused* by the activities or products of a member of the group.

5. The injured person will *release* all participating individuals and organizations from other liability and agree to *resolve all future disputes by arbitration* or other ADR.

6. The offer will be made once there is a *recognition that an infection or injury has occurred*, for example, through the precess of look-back, *or when a claim is brought* against a participant.

7. *Causation will be assumed for certain injuries*, subject to the blood center's or hospital's ability to disprove it, e.g., a known pretransfusion infection or a donor later tests negative.

8. Compensation *funding will be on a pay-as-you-go basis*, with each participant contributing to the pool for its patients.

9. *Allocations of the costs* among the hospital, the blood center, and, where appropriate, the physician will be *negotiated, with a form of ADR* agreed to in advance to resolve disputes.

10. *Claims management*—including both contact with the injured person and management of the claim thereafter—*will be done in a coordinated way* on behalf of all participants.

Although "fault" will be irrelevant to the question of compensation, "causation" will continue to be required. This is an important limitation. Hepatitis is one of the infections that we believe must be among the covered injuries. The prevalence of hepatitis in the general population is so large and so little of it is transfusion related that we must retain the criterion of cause-in-fact to be certain that blood will not carry the insurance premium for all of hepatitis in the patient population regardless of its origin. Given that there is no universal preoperative testing for hepatitis, surrogates for assessing causation will be necessary. If, for example, certain symptoms appear within certain time frames, we will presume causation. The details here are somewhat complex; suffice it to say that they have been worked out to optimize the balance between efficient investigation and accurate compensation.

Once an incident occurs, the patient will be contacted very early on, while the problem is still something that can be managed reasonably and before it becomes an intransigent legal claim. If there are disputes over time as to whether some item of medical expense ought to be covered or not, or whether some portion of a participating person's medical or disability expense falls within the policy, those issues will not be taken back to court but, rather, will be resolved through a private mechanism somewhat resembling arbitration.

The bottom line of the program is that even though more people will be paid something, the efficiencies of running a compensation system in this way are great enough that the program can operate within the existing expenditures for insurance premiums and other payments presently attributable to these same injuries. That, in any event, is the hypothesis that the model is designed to test. Our economic studies suggest that it will work.

The program should be ready by 1996. We have been working on the details of the administrative system, including recruiting additional hospitals and health care providers to the effort. Financially, the system is designed to be at least a break even effort. Compensation efficiency and breadth will be increased, blood centers and hospitals can get out of the litigation business, and compensation for the injured person can be more accurately focused and applied. Finally, this may be a device that has broader application to medical injury generally.

We are of course concerned about whether we did the arithmetic correctly. That is why it is a pilot program. We have put it together with escape valves and brakes that we can apply at any time. We are going to watch it very carefully. But even if it does terminate early, we will guarantee continued benefits to anyone who has already agreed to participate up to that point.

One of the most trenchant criticisms that has been made of this system is what we have been calling the adverse selection effect. Because the offer is made post injury, some observers suggest that all those with currently noneconomic claims will come for the "free money," while those with large, very serious claims will stay in the court system. Thus, it is argued, the program will have the worst of both systems.

We have studied this possibility carefully, and believe that by contrast we may have the best of both systems. There is a substantial advantage to promising to pay a sick person, right now, exactly what is needed, rather than requiring that person to go into a forum in which some may win, most will lose and everyone winds up somewhat worse off. In addition, we have calculated the worst case by assuming that the selection effect does occur and have determined that even if every assumption of the model fails, the outside risk is a manageable one. More realistically, it appears that the process-cost savings from only two court cases avoided will cover the cost of 100 percent of the compensation for injuries not now being paid.

Paul Schmidt: I just paid my $250 to the Florida Neurologic Birth Injury Fund as a pathologist. If I were an obstetrician I would have to pay $5,000. I look at it as the "All babies must be born perfect and all patients must live forever" fund. There was a paper in *Lancet*[108] out of England about 3 months ago looking at hepatitis C in patients in a hematologic, oncologic ward back over the years in which 34 percent of the patients developed hepatitis C. By polymerase chain reaction and other studies it was their opinion that none of the patients got hepatitis C from transfusion. That would be the logical presumption. They were all transfused. They got hepatitis C, but they were convinced that there were other reasons why they got it in the hospital.

Edward A. Dauer: That goes to the question of causation. While we are moving into no-fault, we are not moving into no-cause. One of the things that a patient must establish is that they received a unit of blood that came from one of the participating blood centers. We then do a look-back to see if we can find the donor. There are ways in which we can reduce the probability that payments will be made for hepatitis caused by non-blood components. One of them that has been proposed is that some kinds of symptoms must occur within a certain time frame immediately after the transfusion.

Paul Schmidt: That is based on what we know today, and if we let the science evolve we might find out that it is not the answer. There may be better ways of looking at it.

Edward A. Dauer: We need to make some judgments about what it is we want to accomplish. Over the last 10 years plaintiffs' lawyers have learned how to sue blood banks. They did it with HIV. Hepatitis may well be next.

---

[108] Allander, T, A Gruber, M Naghavi, A Beyene, T Soderstrom, M Bjorkholm, L Grillner, MA Persson (1995). Frequent patient-to-patient transmission of hepatitis C in a haematology ward. *Lancet, 345(8949):* 603–607.

The number of cases we have seen involving plaintiff's actions and hepatitis may be no indication of what we are going to see in the future. We need to make some guesses as to whether this is going to be better or worse.

There are some other interesting pieces of the mathematics. For instance, over 40 percent of all those who receive a transfusion die within a very short time from the underlying condition for which the transfusion was required. We have factored those things in, and the program looks feasible, but it is still a pilot program, and we won't know everything about it until we do it.

William Sherwood: Can you give us some idea of how the compensation works? I gather punitive damages aren't here.

Edward A. Dauer: That is correct.

William Sherwood: Is there pain and suffering?

Edward A. Dauer: No.

William Sherwood: If there are effects with hepatitis or cirrhosis 10 years later, how do those get handled?

Edward A. Dauer: That is precisely what we see as the advantage for those few people who will have serious problems in the future. Under the formal legal system, the statutes of limitations and other rules force people to bring lawsuits before they know the extent of their injuries. What this system would provide to the injured person is a guarantee to cover those needs as they arise in the future. We, in turn, will be working on a funding mechanism to ensure that there is an actuarially appropriate reserve fund or other capability to handle those needs. Coverage of actual medical needs attributable to the injury, to the extent possible under the law, will be in excess of or secondary to existing health care coverage. The details of maintaining an excess position are complex and difficult and, I must say, not yet fully worked out. This is one disadvantage of a private program. However, the program can also be made financially feasible, even if this assumption is incorrect.

The disability loss will be limited to a percentage of the average monthly wage of the average wage earner (plus inflation factors) during that person's working life. We will not pay the lost earnings of a neurosurgeon, for example. This offer, then, might not be as attractive to some people who might be able to do better in court. But we believe a 100 percent probability of meeting one's needs is more attractive than a small probability of achieving one's demands. That is the selling point of this program to the injured people.

It will pay medical expenses and disability as incurred, measured as time goes on, and those funds will be guaranteed through an insurance mechanism.

Henrik Bendixen: You have been explicit about the efficiency achievable with respect to cost. Could you elaborate on the efficiency with respect to time, especially as the court system gets busier and busier?

Edward A. Dauer: That is the reason we think an offer like this makes sense even in the very serious injury case, particularly if someone has a limited life. The process of trial, appeal, and if necessary, retrial can sometimes take longer than the expected life span of the person who has been infected. Our payments will be immediate.

Celso Bianco: There is a lot of resistance to this process in many areas. There is one aspect that the trial lawyers actually play with: the patient's anger and desire for vengeance. How are you going to deal with this?

Edward A. Dauer: There is a growing empirical literature[109] that investigates among people who are injured the question of who brings lawsuits and who doesn't, why they bring lawsuits, and what is it that motivates them. In many ways money is a surrogate for things that don't necessarily require money. In any number of cases dealing with injured neonates we have seen that one of the reasons for a lawsuit was that the parents could not otherwise find out what happened. They brought the lawsuit to go through the formal discovery process and require the physician and the hospital to be forthcoming with information. Our hope is that if people can be dealt with early on in the development of their disappointment, we may be able to satisfy their needs and not have to satisfy many of those demands. Sometimes anger can be dealt with by a $100,000 punitive damages award and sometimes by somebody saying, "I am terribly sorry." The latter is underrated.

Harold Sox: The system that both of you have described appears to deal with the troubles that we know and their actuarial likelihood based on existing resources. Part of the reason that we are here is to anticipate the troubles that we don't know about. Do you have any comments about how that potentiality should be anticipated to develop a better system in the future?

Edward A. Dauer: In doing the calculations as to the cost of this process, we did studies of what the likely known kinds of injuries are going to be. I don't

---

[109] The studies are collected and discussed in chapter 17 of E. Dauer (1994; Suppl. 1995). *Manual of Dispute Resolution: ADR Law and Practice.* Colorado Springs: Shepard's McGraw-Hill.

know how one deals with the cost of unknowns. This program is dealing with cases prospectively only; that is, we are not going to deal with people who have been injured in the past. The reason is that we cannot load onto the present medical system a premium for the accumulated injuries that have occurred up to now. But given a system that only pays damages as they come, there is the opportunity, in effect, to self-insure through the pricing of blood and blood products over a longer period of time that may allow for that adjustment. We are not in the insurance business. What we may find is that reinsurance of the guarantees will require an insurer to do that additional prognostication. We don't know how to do that directly.

Mason Howard: The issues in blood products are a little bit different from those in all the rest of medical practice. I cannot answer how you address something that is going to appear in the future. I do believe, however, that with the system that we propose there will be an enhanced level of provider behavior in our state because of the system. I hope there will also be a better level of practice because of loss control activities that are focused right where the injuries are occurring.

William Sherwood: Blood banking might be a small pool where a major disaster, such as AIDS, hits it disproportionately compared with the rest of the health care system. If there were a larger pool, such as more of the health care system, over which to distribute the potential risks, would that be a better scenario?

Edward A. Dauer: That would be very nice, but it may not be feasible just yet. We have achieved in our project the cooperation of hospitals that are very interested in the no-fault idea and in taking a share of the expenses to evaluate the model. They want to see how this works in a limited area like blood before moving toward doing something similar to cover other areas of medical injury. On the other hand, the hospital community may still be hoping that a resolution of the malpractice problem will be forthcoming from the legislatures. Apart from no-fault programs such as those proposed for Colorado and Utah—which offer a trade, essentially, of no-fault liability for limited economic recovery—I would not bet very much on any major legislative reduction in the liability picture in the near future.

VII

Concluding Remarks

Henrik H. Bendixen

Chair, Forum on Blood Safety and Blood Availability

As we review the risks of transfusion, as well as the perception of risk expressed by recipients and the public at large, we should examine all data and all issues in the context of health care and society at large. Since World War II the growth in knowledge and technology has been amazing, leading to substantial advances in safety, including the safety of the blood supply. One important development is the growing importance of computers and information systems. These increasingly drive the way we do research, teach, and train, as well as every aspect of health care practice.

During the same period of time, public attitudes have changed from the acceptance of a tragic mishap as an act of God to today's unwillingness to accept anything other than a perfect result. We do not know all the reasons why this change is taking place, but attitudes certainly have changed, irreversibly, and we see this change in attitude reflected in everything from legislation and regulation to accreditation requirements, lawsuits, and the media.

Returning to the advances in the safety of the blood supply, we must observe that a finite risk remains, a risk that may or may not be acceptable. What are the factors that influence the degree of acceptability or lack of acceptability of a given risk? First, there is informed consent. Granger Morgan's presentation on risk communication stressed how informed consent converts an involuntary risk into a voluntarily acceptable risk, provided the consent is competently obtained. In Nelson's study of patients undergoing open heart surgery, the patients gave informed consent not only to the surgery but also to receiving multiple blood transfusions. The risk of multiple transfusions was not trivial, yet it was acceptable, being relatively small compared with the risks of surgery, anesthesia, and the heart disease itself. Sometimes informed consent cannot be obtained, such as in major trauma, and while the risk of transfusion may still be modest compared with the total risk, it is still an involuntary risk. Finally, when transfusion of blood or a blood product stands alone as the only intervention, that is when the risk is least acceptable, particularly when it is unknown and therefore not voluntarily accepted.

Moreno recommended that we err on the side of hyperinforming in obtaining informed consent. He presented a tiered process, starting with a relatively concise explanation and moving on to an explicit invitation to the patient to ask questions. A second tier would be to respond to any questions that are asked, while a third tier might be to provide written material or references.

The conflict between individual rights, placing autonomy first, and the needs and financial concerns of society at large will always be with us. Fiscal realities will drive us to find rationales within our liberal framework to explain where we draw the limits on the share of common resources that the individual can claim. We are groping toward an adaptation of public philosophy to real-world constraints. The Oregon experience of having panels of experts rank treatments and procedures according to both benefit and cost is an intriguing program. Community groups then did their independent ranking, which, at least in part, was different from that of the experts, but the result was a plan that had community support. The result of involving the community as decision makers was building trust.

The concept of informed consent goes beyond the specific consent obtained for a specific procedure to the acceptance of patients' right to know and to be active decision makers about their own health or illness. The loss of trust referred to by Chess could have been avoided or mitigated had those at greatest risk been active participants in the decision-making process during the early days of the HIV problem. The vice chairman of the National Hemophilia Foundation reminded the Forum of the importance of trust and its enhancement by open communication.

Many factors have contributed to improved blood safety, including new concepts, good research, ever better technology, and computer-based quality control. Also contributing have been the introduction of guidelines and standards by professional groups, as well as the influence of the press, consumer groups, special interest groups, and even lawsuits. Regulations by federal or state agencies have played a special role. Advances in safety, however, do not logically argue for deregulation, but in a modern industrial society, one important facilitator is "predictability." There must be some rules of the game, and one can accept even tough rules, as long as they are well known and equitably administered. Much has been learned from more than 10 years of dealing with HIV in the blood supply, and much progress has been made. All of that knowledge should help us in preparing for the defense against the next new illness to descend upon us.

Appendixes

A

Acronyms and Abbreviations

AABB	American Association of Blood Banks
ADR	alternative dispute resolution
AHCPR	Agency for Health Care Policy and Research
AHF	antihemophilic factor
AIDS	acquired immunodeficiency syndrome
ALS	amyotrophic lateral sclerosis
ALT	alanine aminotransferase
ARC	American Red Cross
CAT	computer assisted tomography
CCBC	Council of Community Blood Centers
CDC	Centers for Disease Control and Prevention
CFU	colony forming unit
CJD	Creutzfeldt-Jakob disease
CMV	cytomegalovirus
CNS	central nervous system
CPR	Center for Public Resources
DNA PCR	deoxyribonucleic acid polymerase chain reaction
EIS	Epidemic Intelligence Service
ELISA I/II	Enzyme-linked immunosorbent assay I/II
EPA	Environmental Protection Agency
FACTS	Frequency of Agents Communicable by Transfusion Study
FDA	Food and Drug Administration
FFP	fresh frozen plasma
GLPR	General Leukocyte and Plasma Repository
GSR	General Serum Repository

HAM/TSP	HTLV-associated myelopathy/tropical spastic paraparesis
HAV	hepatitis A virus
HBsAg	hepatitis B surface antigen
HBV	hepatitis B virus
HCFA	Health Care Financing Administration
HCV	hepatitis C virus
Hgb	hemoglobin
HIV	human immunodeficiency virus
HMO	health maintenance organization
HRSA	Health Resources and Services Administration
HTLV I/II	Human T-lymphotropic virus I/II
ICL	idiopathic CD4 lymphocytopenia
IOM	Institute of Medicine
IRB	institutional review board
MMWR	*Morbidity an Mortality Weekly Report*
MRI	magnetic resonance imaging
NHF	National Hemophilia Foundation
NHLBI	National Heart, Lung and Blood Institute
NIH	National Institutes of Health
PFU	plaque forming unit
PHA	phytohemagglutinin
RBCC	red blood cell concentrate
REDS	Retrovirus Epidemiology of Donors Study
RIBA	radioimmunoblot assay
RNA PCR	ribonucleic acid polymerase chain reaction
S/D	solvent/detergent
TB	tuberculosis
TNBP	tri(n-butyl)phosphate
TTV	transfusion-transmitted virus
UBS	United Blood Services
UVA	ultraviolet A (light)
UVC	ultraviolet C (light)
VSV	vesicular stomatitis virus

B

Workshop Participants

WORKSHOP ON BLOOD BANK OPERATIONS
July 23–24, 1994

James B. AuBuchon, M.D.
Medical Director
Department of Pathology
Dartmouth-Hitchcock Medical Center

Jay Epstein, M.D.
Center for Biologics Evaluation
   and Research
Food and Drug Administration

William Andrew Heaton, M.D.
Irwin Memorial Blood Center

Paul Holland, M.D.
Director
Sacramento Medical Foundation

P. Ann Hoppe
Assistant to the Director
Office of Blood Research and Review
Food and Drug Administration

Claude Lenfant, M.D.
Director
National Heart, Lung and Blood Institute

James MacPherson
Executive Director
Council of Community Blood Centers

Herb Perkins
Irwin Memorial Blood Center

James Reilly
Executive Director
American Blood Resources Association

Jenni Lee Robins
Director, Total Quality Management
New York Blood Center

George B. Schreiber, D.Sc.
Westat, Inc.

Ernest R. Simon, M.D.
Executive Vice President
Scientific, Medical and Technical Affairs
Blood Systems, Inc.

Edwin A. Steane, Ph.D.
Principal Officer
American Red Cross Blood Services

Charles Wallas, M.D.
Director, Blood Bank
Vanderbilt University Medical Center

WORKSHOP ON RISK AND REGULATION
January 23–24, 1995

Lew Barker
Efficacy Trials Branch
Vaccine and Prevention Research
 Program
Division of AIDS, NIAID, NIH

Celso Bianco, M.D.
Vice President, Medical Affairs
New York Blood Center

Penny Chan, Ph.D.
Commission of Inquiry
Blood Systems in Canada
Toronto, Ontario

Harry W. Chen
HemaSure Inc.
Marlborough, MA

Eileen Church
Communications Manager
American Association of Blood Banks

Marcia Crosse
Program Evaluation and Methodology
 Division
U.S. General Accounting Office

Jacqueline D'Alessio, Ph.D.
U.S. General Accounting Office

Leonard I. Friedman
American Red Cross
Holland Lab

Elizabeth Goss
Fox, Bennett & Turner
Washington, DC

Harold Kaplan, M.D.
University of Texas
Southwestern Medical Center

Kurt R. Kroemer
U.S. General Accounting Office

Jan Lane
American Red Cross

Karen Shoos Lipton
CEO
American Association of Blood Banks

Jane Mackey, MBA
Topeka Blood Bank, Inc.

James MacPherson
Executive Director
Council of Community Blood Centers

John McCray
HemaSure Inc.
Marlborough, MA

Brian McDonough
American Red Cross
Arlington, VA

Charles Mosher
Blood Centers of America, Inc.
East Greenwich, RI

Jean Otter
Director of Regulatory Affairs
American Association of Blood Banks

Mary K. Pendergast
Deputy Commissioner and
 Senior Advisor to the Commissioner
Food and Drug Administration

Barbara Peoples
American Red Cross
Holland Lab

APPENDIX B

Mark Philip
IMMUNO US, Inc.
Rochester, MI

Beatrice Pierce
National Hemophilia Foundation
Rancho Santa Fe, CA

William H. Portman
The Institute for Transfusion Medicine
Pittsburgh, PA

James Reilly
Executive Director
American Blood Resources Association

Miriam Sparrow, Esq.
New York Blood Center, Inc.

Edwin Steane, Ph.D.
ICCBBA

Eugene Timm
IMMUNO US, Inc.
Rochester, MI

Peter Tomasulo, M.D.
TM Consulting, Inc.
McLean, VA

Lee Ann Weitekamp
The Blood Center of Southeastern Wisconsin
Milwaukee, WI

WORKSHOP ON MANAGING THREATS TO THE BLOOD SUPPLY
September 21–22, 1995

Lew Barker
Efficacy Trials Branch
Vaccine and Prevention Research Program
Division of AIDS, NIAID, NIH

Patricia Bezjak
Chief Operating Officer
Metropolitan Washington Blood Banks

Celso Bianco, M.D.
Vice President, Medical Affairs
New York Blood Center

Eileen Church
Communications Manager
American Association of Blood Banks

Brian P. Conway, Esq.
Bayer Corporation

Richard J. Davey, M.D.
Chief Medical Officer
American Red Cross

Rob Dickstein
Director, Regulatory Affairs
Pall Corporation

Sandra Ellisor
Ortho Diagnostic Systems, Inc.

Susan Frantz-Bohn
Division of Congressional and Public Affairs
Center for Biologics Research and Evaluation
Food and Drug Administration

Steve Friedman
Dechert, Price, & Rhoads

Eric Goosby
Office of HIV/AIDS Policy
Public Health Service

Elizabeth Goss
Fox, Bennett & Turner
Washington, DC

William J. Hammes
Associate Counsel
Bayer Corporation

Harriet Newman, (MT) ASCP
Donor Advocate
Virginia Blood Services

Nancy Newman
Knapp, Petersen & Clark

Jean Otter
Director of Regulatoy Affairs
American Association of Blood Banks

Stephen Redhead
Congressional Research Service
Library of Congress

James Reilly
Executive Director
American Blood Resources Association

Paul Schmidt, M.D.
Head, Transfusion Medicine
Transfusion Medicine Academic Center
Florida Blood Services

Toby Simon, M.D.
President and CEO
Blood Systems, Inc.

Harold C. Sox, Jr., M.D.
Chairman, Department of Medicine
Dartmouth-Hitchcock Medical Center

Miriam Sparrow, Esq.
New York Blood Center, Inc.

Jane Starkey
Deputy Director
Council of Community Blood Centers

Ron Welborn
Community Bioresources, Inc.

Edward Wolf
Senior Associate General Council
American Red Cross

Sam Wortham
Group Vice President
Pall Corporation